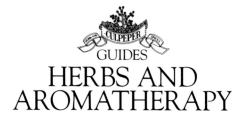

GUIDES

HERBS AND
AROMATHERAPY

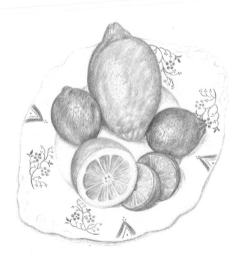

Grapefruit, orange and tangerine

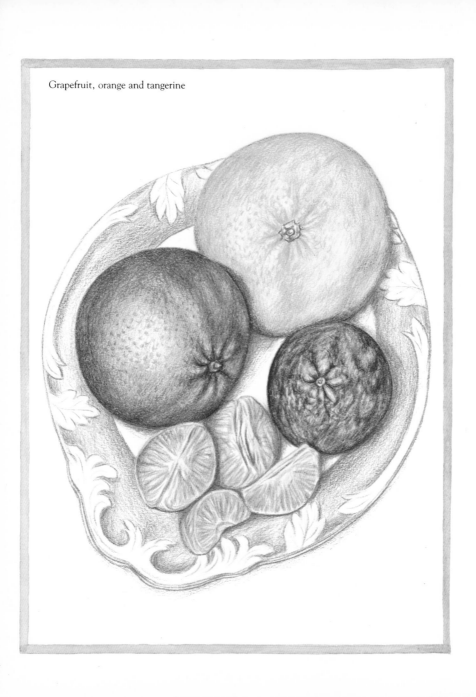

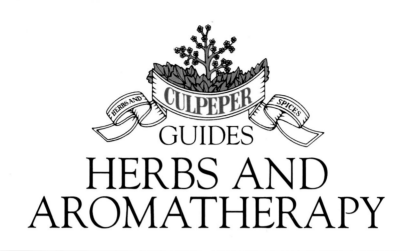

GUIDES
HERBS AND
AROMATHERAPY

JOANNAH METCALFE

Illustrated by
ROSAMUND GENDLE

General Editor
IAN THOMAS

Bloomsbury Books
London

Half title: Lemon and lime

First published in Great Britain 1989 by
Webb & Bower (Publishers) Limited

This edition published 1993 by
Bloomsbury Books an imprint of
Godfrey Cave Associates
42 Bloomsbury Street, London WC1B 3QJ
under license from Webb & Bower Ltd.

ISBN I-85471-072-9

Designed by Ron Pickless

Production by Nick Facer/Rob Kendrew

Illustrations by Rosamund Gendle

General Editor Ian Thomas

Text Copyright © 1989 Joannah Metcalfe
Culpeper Trade Mark Copyright © 1989 Culpeper Limited
Design and layout Copyright © 1989 Webb & Bower (Publishers) Limited

Printed in Italy by A. Pizzi, Milan

Typeset in Great Britain by P&M Typesetting, Exeter, Devon

CONTENTS

Author's Note

It is important to note that this book serves as an introduction to and description of aromatherapy. Those readers who are interested in taking the matter further should refer to the reference books listed in the appendix, and to the International Federation of Aromatherapists (IFA).

It must be strongly emphasized that any reader tempted to use essential oils not described in this book should refrain from doing so, without further reference to or advice from an IFA accredited aromatherapist. These essential oils may prove harmful, as there are a number of oils which are known to be toxic and should not be used under any circumstances.

On a final note, it is interesting to consider the few species of plants that have been the subject of research, producing the relatively small amount of essential oils currently available. Who can say what benefit has already been lost as a result of the destruction of the world's natural resources, especially the rain forests. We must do all we can to promote both conservation and research so that aromatherapy and other valuable therapies can be re-enforced and extended, for the benefit of both this and future generations.

AROMATHERAPY

WHAT IS IT?

Aromatherapy involves the use of essential oils to promote and maintain health and vitality. These essences are extracted from aromatic plants, flowers and trees. The properties of these oils, and their lack of side-effects when used correctly, make aromatherapy a viable alternative and addition to orthodox treatment for many conditions.

The oils are used in many forms: massage, inhalations, aromatic baths, compresses, cosmetic preparations and many other specific applications. Due to the extreme concentration of plant material in each essential oil droplet, essential oils are invariably diluted before use, and must be used with great care.

HOW DO THE OILS WORK?

Scientific research is constantly producing more information on the action of essential oils, and many more wonderful secrets are undoubtedly awaiting discovery. We know that there are three basic routes by which the oils are absorbed into the system.

During inhalations and massage the vapours are inhaled. The lungs are lined with a rich blood supply which readily absorbs the essential oil molecules. These then travel around the body for several hours before they are eliminated. The skin also absorbs the essences. During massage, the diluted blend of essence and vegetable oil is absorbed into the blood stream through the pores in the skin. A uniform absorption takes place during a full body massage as the essences travel into the interstitial fluid between each cell.

The actions of the essences then vary according to their constituents. Some stimulate our circulation, increasing the rate of elimination of toxic substances such as uric acid. Other oils act on specific organs, increasing their secretions of body chemicals such as the production of bile by the liver, or oestrogen by the ovaries. The majority are highly antiseptic, and thus extremely useful in the treatment of infections. Many essences also have an analgesic effect, and the aromatherapy treatment can stimulate the release of endorphins – body chemicals which have a pain-killing and anti-depressant effect.

Most essential oils have a specific effect on the emotional as well as the physical level. As the vapours are inhaled impulses pass along the olfactory nerve from the nasal cavity, which is connected to the limbic system in the brain. This is the part of the brain that deals with memory and emotion. Certain oils then stimulate specific neuro-chemicals within the nervous system. Sedative oils such as lavender and marjoram stimulate the neuro-chemical serotonin, which induces sleep. These oils therefore have a calming, sedating effect and can, for instance, be used to treat tension and insomnia.

These examples demonstrate how the diverse actions of the essences have far-reaching and wide-ranging actions. Holistic aromatherapy, by restoring and promoting the balance between body and mind, can help prevent illness. If illness or mechanical damage occur, aromatherapy then stimulates the body's ability to help itself.

DIFFERENT FORMS OF AROMATHERAPY
Although essential oils have been used for at least five thousand years, aromatherapy today is still undergoing the process of rediscovery and evolution. I myself promote the use of the oils in a holistic fashion, and underline the necessity for adequate knowledge of these powerful substances, to prevent misuse.

The following categories outline the basic forms of aromatherapy:

1 Clinical aromatherapy
This involves using the oils internally, taking tiny prescribed dilutions orally. Some French doctors trained in aromatherapy practise this method but it is **not** recommended for home use.

WARNING: **Do not take any essential oils orally without qualified medical supervision.**

2 Holistic aromatherapy
This form of treatment should be practised by well-trained practitioners (see IFA Accredited Schools). The initial consultation should involve talking through medical history, diet, exercise, general life-style and any problems encountered. The

whole person should be taken into account, not just one specific symptom.

3 Aromatherapy and (aesthetic aromatherapy) beauticians

Many beauty therapists now include essences in treatment oils, creams and lotions, to be used on a superficial level, primarily for skin treatment. Many of the essences have an extremely beneficial action on the skin, and this form of treatment can be both pleasant and rewarding. The knowledge involved should not however be confused with the holistic healing treatment. Many people mistakenly believe that aromatherapy is basically a beauty treatment. This is only one of the many facets that aromatherapy treatment has to offer.

WHY AROMATHERAPY?

Why has aromatherapy recently become so popular? There has been a general upsurge of interest in holistic medicine of different types. Herbalism, acupuncture, homoeopathy; these therapies and others aim at treating the whole person using remedies which are free from harmful side-effects, and help to prevent the symptoms of 'disease'.

Holistic aromatherapy combines both an extremely enjoyable treatment and 'self-help' advice which constitutes an effective therapy in its own right. The many factors that combine to lower our quality of life, and ultimately our state of health, can often be tackled by holistic aromatherapy, by rebalancing the system and restoring homoeostasis (see diagram on page 10).

Obviously the diagram is an over simplification of what leads to illness. Aromatherapy is not a 'cure all' either! But the illustration is generally appropriate for most people and the majority of diseases. The vicious circle that leads to illness can be identified by us all. It is no coincidence that we get a cold when we can least afford the time or energy to deal with it! Neither is it surprising that when we are 'down' emotionally, everything seems to go wrong, for this is the time when our immune system becomes less effective, and we are more open to the adverse effects of our environment and life-style.

We are very sensitive tactile creatures; we need human contact. Massage is an instinctive reaction. When we bang ourselves, we rub the area to ease the pain; we comfort a child by a hug and a cuddle. As we mature, the physical contact diminishes, and yet general pressures often increase. The compassionate impartial massage relieves muscular spasm, re-educating the muscles, enabling us to achieve a more relaxed posture. The circulation is stimulated, increasing the rate of toxin removal. Problems may be shared, and pressures eased. General peace of mind is promoted.

The merit of such treatment and the use of essential oils in the home cannot be over emphasized.

NEGATIVE CYCLE
LEADING TO ILLNESS

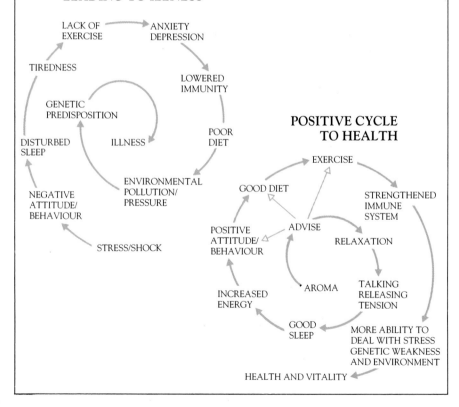

ESSENTIAL AND BASE OILS

WHAT IS AN ESSENTIAL OIL?

An essential oil is a highly concentrated aromatic substance which evaporates easily. It is extracted by distillation or expression from a single source. This may be any species of:

Flower	Seed
Fruit (peel)	Root
Grass	Tree
Leaf	

HOW ARE THEY EXTRACTED?

There are three methods involved in the extraction of these essences:
1 Distillation
2 Expression
3 Solvent extraction

1 Distillation

The majority of true essences are distilled in the following way: large vats are filled with plant material which is steamed at a high pressure. The steam and essential oil vapour is then cooled, condensed and collected.

2 Expression

The citrus oils are obtained by simply expressing – (squeezing) the fruit peel, which contains the essential oil droplets. Lemon, lime, mandarin, orange and bergamot are all obtained in this way.

3 Solvent extraction

When flowers, such as rose and jasmine, are delicate, the heat and pressure used in distillation would evaporate the oil molecules, which would subsequently be lost. Therefore the following expensive and relatively time-consuming process is particularly important: the solvents benzene, butane, alcohol or luxane are used. Many tonnes of flowers are macerated and soaked in one of the solvents. The mixture is then centrifuged to separate the oils and waxes from the solvent and waste material. The 'concrete' of oils and waxes is then distilled in a vacuum, which can take place at a very low temperature. The wax is separated from the absolute, the final result.

WHERE TO BUY AND HOW TO STORE QUALITY ESSENTIAL AND BASE OILS

Buying essential oils

There is currently considerable confusion when it comes to buying good-quality essential oils. How do we ascertain the standards of purity and quality? These are some basic rules to remember:

1 If they are labelled 'aromatherapy oils' or any description other than 'pure essential oil' it is unlikely that they are pure essences. They will probably contain a high percentage of vegetable or mineral oil to 'stretch' the pure essential oil. The therapeutic properties will therefore be greatly reduced.

2 True essential oils are often expensive. Some of the basic (and versatile) essences such as lavender, tea-tree and the citrus oils can be produced reasonably inexpensively, and their cost should therefore reflect this. The oils of rose, jasmine, neroli and others come from delicate flowers. The extraction process is an expensive one, and the price will be concomitantly high. If it is not, they will be not pure essences.

3 Some therapists may charge excessively high prices for essential oils, as they may order in small amounts. This must also be taken into consideration.

4 Essential oils should be sold in dark glass bottles. This again may be an indication of purity and quality, for if the oils have been kept in clear glass or plastic the light may have detrimentally affected them. A reputable dealer will be aware of this.

Buying base oils

The best quality, vegetable base (or carrier) oils are obtained by 'cold-pressing'. This means that the almonds, for instance, have been crushed to express the oil, which has then been drained off and filtered. The 'virgin' oil is the highest quality and comes from the first pressing. It contains the highest vitamin and mineral content, and has been produced by natural means.

After the first pressing, the process then involves other lesser quality production. This uses heat, and the oil may be treated synthetically to deodorize, remove colour, or obtain other such results. The vitamin and mineral content will be drastically reduced during these processes.

The best base oils will therefore be labelled 'cold-pressed', and often 'virgin' too. Most will have a rich colour and a characteristic aroma.

It is therefore recommended to buy your essential and base oils from a reputable company such as Culpeper (which also has a mail-order service). You can then dilute and blend them yourself (see Recipes, page 88). Then you will be sure of the products you use, and the percentage dilution at which you use them.

How to store essential and base oils

Both essential and vegetable base oils will need to be stored in the right conditions to keep well. They react to strong sunlight, oxygen and heat. They should be kept in dark glass bottles (essential oils will corrode plastic) in a dry, cool, dark place. Most have a longer 'shelf life' when stored separately, so the blend of essential oils in vegetable oil should be made up in relatively small amounts, and used accordingly.

The average shelf life for an essential oil is two years. The more often the oil is used, the more quickly the oxygen in the air combines with certain constituents in the oil to oxidize it. When this happens, the therapeutic effect of the oil gradually diminishes and the aroma will be altered. The oil will eventually go cloudy, a sign that it has 'gone off'.

Citrus essences have the shorter shelf life of six months, as they have a high proportion (approximately 90%) of limonene. This is a terpene which combines with oxygen very readily. Thus grapefruit, lemon, mandarin and the other citrus essences should only be bought in small quantities. Bergamot is an exception here, and will store well. Neroli will last approximately one year.

The vegetable oils will also 'go off' for the same reason, as oxidization takes place. They will go cloudy and smell rancid. Wheatgerm and avocado oils last the longest due to their high vitamin E content. (They can be added to a blend, especially one containing citrus essences, to prolong shelf life.)

Some essential oils, notably the thicker essences extracted from trees (gums and resins) will last much longer than the average essence if stored correctly – up to five years or even longer. A few essences, such as patchouli and myrrh actually improve with age.

SOME DEFINITIONS
An infused oil
This method of using essential oil was first used by ancient civilizations thousands of years ago. A vegetable base oil has plant material added and is heated, or left in the sun. The vegetable oil absorbs the essential constituents of the plant material. Calendula oil and comfrey oil are examples.

(It is impossible to make your own essential oils. This is due to the enormous amount of plant material needed to make each drop of essence. It is possible to make infused oils in the house. This can be both enjoyable and rewarding. See Recipes, page 88.)

Aromatic chemical
Each constituent of essential oil is an aromatic chemical. There are many synthetic counterparts which are used in the manufacture of modern perfumes and cosmetics.

Perfume
Ancient perfumes consisted almost entirely of aromatic essences. Modern man uses synthetic aromatic chemicals to produce the large amounts of perfumes and cosmetics people now demand. Some of the more expensive perfumes contain up to 20% of essential oil. (The ancient perfumes must have imparted a therapeutic effect as well as an amazing aroma!)

IMPORTANT POINTS TO REMEMBER WHEN USING ESSENTIAL OILS
1 Each drop of essential oil is extremely concentrated and should be used with great care.

2 Only lavender and tea-tree may be used undiluted in small amounts. No other essence should be used undiluted.

3 Certain emmenagogic essences (those that stimulate oestrogen production) and generally stimulatory oils should **not be used during pregnancy**. This is especially important during the first three months, and for those with a fragile pregnancy. These essences may stimulate menstrual bleeding, causing abortion.

4 Babies and children have very delicate, sensitive skins. They are inclined to rub their eyes and suck fingers in the bath. Essences should therefore be diluted at quarter the adult strength, and diluted again before adding to the bath.

5 Great care should be taken to avoid getting essential oils in the eye, as this can cause permanent damage. If it does happen, wash out the eye with water and consult a doctor immediately.

6 Never leave young children alone with a bowl of hot water that is being used for an inhalation. Always ensure there is adult supervision at all times, and give inhalations for a short time only.

7 Always keep the eyes closed during the use of essential oil inhalations.

8 It is advisable to dilute essential oils in a small amount of vegetable oil or full fat (not skimmed milk) before adding to the bath and to agitate the water. This ensures the essence is uniformly dispersed, and does not cause irritation.

9 Never use more than 10 drops of essential oil in the bath.

10 Never use higher than a 2.5% dilution of essence unless under professional instruction.

11 Never give or take essence orally (by mouth).

12 Those with very sensitive skin may find it prudent to use a 1% dilution of essential oil to help prevent an allergic reaction. It is also advisable to avoid any oils which are possible skin irritants (see appendix). Try the skin patch technique before more general use of the oil (see page 16).

13 Always consult a medically qualified practitioner in the event of serious illness, or worsening condition. This is especially important where children are concerned, and in cases of high temperatures, convulsions and bad burns.

If in doubt, consult your medical practitioner

SKIN PATCH TEST

1 Prepare and blend the oils you wish to test.
2 Wash and dry the forearm thoroughly.
3 Apply droplets of the blend on to the gauze section of a large plaster. The pad should be completely saturated with the oil (but not to the extent that seepage occurs).
4 Place the plaster on the forearm, and leave in place for 24 hours. Remove immediately if irritation or sensitization occurs.
5 Remove plaster after the 24-hour period, and examine the area of skin in contact with the gauze. If the area is very red, irritated or sensitive DO NOT USE the proposed blend. If the area appears normal, proceed as planned.

NOTE: This basic skin patch test does not guarantee that there will be no adverse reaction. It will help determine those essential oils which do not suit certain skin types.

CARRIER/BASE OILS

The use of high-quality vegetable oils in aromatherapy is obviously very important, for the following reasons:
1 They provide a natural medium in which the essential oils can be diluted without harmfully altering their therapeutic effect.
2 The vegetable oil molecules are absorbed into the blood-stream through the skin pores, unlike mineral oils. The essential oils are also absorbed in the vegetable blend, and can therefore have the desired action.
3 The nutritional constituents of the vegetable oils (such as vitamins A and E) nourish the skin itself.
4 The oil acts as a lubricant between hand and skin in massage, allowing the hands to glide over the skin easily.

Many of the richer, thicker oils, such as wheatgerm and avocado, are most useful when diluted in a 'universal' base such as sweet almond, soya, sunflower or grapeseed oil. All these are easily absorbed by the skin, while the thicker oils are heavier and sticky.

The quality of the oils is important. The more highly processed the vegetable oils are, the less vitamin content will be retained. The best quality oils are therefore those which have been cold-pressed, (preferably the 'virgin' type) and untreated by chemicals.

Once opened and exposed to the oxygen in the air, vegetable oils will last up to six months. They should be kept in the fridge and discarded if the mild characteristic smell begins to turn rancid, and the clear oil becomes cloudy. Always store in clean airtight containers.

(NOTE: If storing your vegetable oil in the fridge, remember to remove well before use in massage. Cold oil is not condusive to relaxation!)

Avocado oil
A thick, heavy oil, this makes a useful addition to many blends, adding a rich green colour. This oil also helps preserve the blend, due to a high vitamin E content. It also contains vitamin A, which makes it especially useful for skin problems. It is safe to use for those suffering from wheat allergies. Due to its thick consistency and high vitamin content, it should generally be used in a 5% dilution.

Evening primrose oil
This is expressed from the seeds of *Oenothera biennis*, a tall plant with pretty yellow flowers attractive to bees. This oil is used internally in capsule form for skin conditions, pre-menstrual tension and the early stages of multiple sclerosis. It is thus a useful addition to treatment oils for eczema and other dry skin conditions. It is soothing and healing for inflammatory allergic conditions.

Jojoba 'oil'
This is derived from a desert plant *Simmondsia chinensis*. It is a diluted wax which gives the skin a wonderfully silky feel and adds extra fluidity for a massage blend; use at 10% dilution. This is particularly useful for dry eczema. (Jojoba is the plant substitute for an extract taken from the intestines of sperm whales.)

Peach and apricot kernel oils
These are expressed from the kernels of *Prunus persica* (peach kernel oil is otherwise known as persic oil) and *Prunus armenica*.

The oils have very little aroma, and have similar qualities to almond oil. (All these are basically inexpensive.)

Soya oil
This oil has emollient properties and is used in the treatment of dry skin in bath preparations and massage. It is specifically useful for those who have an allergic reaction to wheatgerm and dairy products.

Sweet almond oil
Sweet almond oil has a characteristic smell, and is cold-pressed from the seeds of the sweet almond. It is pale yellow, and contains the glycerides of oleic, linoleic and palmitic acids. It has emollient, softening and nutritive qualities.

Wheatgerm oil
This is a very rich nourishing oil, which adds a beautiful orange colour to your blend. It is extremely useful, as it has a high vitamin E content. This is very good for the skin, especially dry, cracked or mature skin. It helps prevent stretch marks and generally soothes and heals. It makes a useful addition to most **blends** of bath oils and skin preparations. Vitamin E also preserves the life of the blend as it has an anti-oxidant effect. It should be used in the treatment of skin conditions. Generally, it is more useful as an addition to another base oil, at about 10%.

CAUTION: **Wheatgerm oil may irritate the skin of anyone with a wheat allergy.**

General base oils
The choice of the base oil to which the aforementioned oils and essences will be added is really a matter of personal preference or therapeutic needs. Sweet almond oil is a general favourite. It has a pleasing and mild fragrance, is easily absorbed by the skin and is not too thick or sticky.

The main points to remember when choosing your base oil are:
- Quality (cold-pressed)
- Texture (sticky or fluid)

- Absorbability
- Fragrance (olive oil can impart an unpleasant undesirable odour)

Oils recommended as general base oils are:
Sweet almond
Peach kernel
Apricot kernel
Grapeseed
Sunflower seed
Sesame seed
Soya bean oil

Diluting and blending essential oils

There are many differing opinions as to the amount of essential oil to use in each blend, and the number of essences that should be combined for maximum therapeutic effect. I must therefore emphasize the fact that the following recommendations are my own personal preference. I was taught to use the essences in this manner by Mike Dowling, Maria Raworth and Robert Tisserand. Together, these people represent years of experience in the world of aromatherapy.

It is recommended that a 2½% concentration is used for a basic dilution. This is a lot easier than it sounds!

Step 1
Ascertain the size of the bottle in mililitres (ml). This will be stamped on the bottom or on the label if the bottle is second-hand (if neither, fill the bottle with water, pour into a measuring jug and read off the measurement).

Step 2
Having ascertained the volume, halve the number to give the correct number of drops to add; this will achieve the desired concentration of 2½%.

EXAMPLE
50ml (2fl oz/¼ cup) bottle – 25 drops
30ml (1fl oz/2tbs) bottle – 15 drops   } 2½%
10ml (¼fl oz/1tbs) bottle – 5 drops

Step 3
One essence may be added to the vegetable oil, or a blend of essences may be added. If this is required, two or three essences are usually sufficient to provide a pleasing aroma and a good therapeutic effect (more than five essences in a blend may begin to counteract the effect!).

If mixing a strong oil (such as eucalyptus) with a weaker one (such as lavender), use three drops of the weak oil to every one drop of the strong. If using oils of similar strength, use the same amount of each. Do this until the correct number of drops are obtained, and a reasonably balanced aroma should be the result. Do not use more essence than the number suggested by the above method, remember how strong they are. Use fewer drops if so desired.

Good results are obtained with practice and familiarity with the oils. If difficulty or confusion results, do not worry. There are many recipes in Chapter 8 covering a wide range of bath oils, facial preparations, inhalations and other specific applications.

It is recommended that preparations for children and those with sensitive skins should be of a 1% concentration.

EXAMPLE:
1¼% dilution is obtained by halving the 2½% method.

50ml (2fl oz/¼ cup) bottle → ½ 25 drops = 12½ (12)
12 drops per 50ml of oil will be approx 1%

30ml (1fl oz/2tbs) bottle → ½ 15 drops = 7½ (7)
7 drops per 30ml = approx 1%

10ml (¼fl oz/1tbs) bottle → 2½ drops of essence = approx 1%

Therapeutic use of essential and base oils
There is such a wide variety of methods in which the essences can be put to use. Just as the properties and actions of these oils vary, so does the way in which they can be used. (See Chapter 8 for recipes.)

Hair treatment/scalp tonic
Problems such as dry hair, dandruff, greasy hair and even hair lice respond well to specific blends of essences diluted in a vegetable oil. Not only are these treatments completely natural (thus useful for those who react allergically to strong perfumes and chemicals in many conditions) but they impart a glorious scent too!

Facial creams, toners, lotions and specific treatment preparations
For general skin care and skin problems, the essences have a variety of qualities of extreme value. Lavender, neroli, patchouli and others are cytophylactc (they stimulate normal skin growth) and have a rejuvenating effect on the skin.

Most of the essences are antiseptic and are therefore used to treat spots and any skin problems associated with infection. Many essences have an astringent cleansing effect and can be included in lotions to cleanse oily skins.

The soothing inflammatory action of oils such as rose and neroli have an excellent action on sensitive skins and cypress, sandalwood and neroli help treat broken veins.

The high vitamin E and A content of vegetable oils such as wheatgerm and avocado make a useful addition to preparations for mature, cracked or dry skin. Problems such as cold sores, eczema, psoriasis and oral thrush also respond extremely well to specific treatment applied to the areas concerned.

It must be emphasized that general aromatherapy treatment will also improve skin tone, stimulating circulation and toxin removal, relieving stress and balancing the system.

Inhalation, mouthwash and gargles
For respiratory problems and general infection, this is an ideal way of introducing the essences into the blood stream. They will then stimulate the body's defence mechanisms and help kill the invading bacteria, virus or fungi. Respiratory infections respond very well, as the heat of the steam acts on the area of infection, as well as on the essences. Many have an expectorant and analgesic effect too.

Gargles can be used to help fight infection and mouthwashes will act on mouth ulcers, oral thrush and infected gums.

Massage oils
This application can be blended to suit all manner of problems, from muscular aches and pains, to skin conditions, to emotional anxiety and tension. Essential oils are diluted in vegetable base oils for this purpose.

Aromatic baths
Bath oils are an important aspect of aromatherapy for health and beauty. They can be stimulating and refreshing for the morning, or relaxing and sedating for sleeping problems. They can be detoxifying, regenerating or comforting. The essential oils are added to a vegetable base. This is added to the bath water, which should then be agitated by hand to disperse the droplets.

Sitz/hip baths
These are especially useful for genito-urinary infections such as thrush, or for use in speeding up the healing process after childbirth.

Essential oil 'burner', diffuser or spray
Different forms of these can be bought in health-food shops, mail-order catalogues, or made up from plant sprays. They are used as a safe, natural ozone friendly way of freshening a room or aiding sleep. They can also be useful during illness – an anti-bacterial spray will kill airborne bacteria and help prevent the spread of infection. Diffusing oils such as eucalyptus will help ease congestion during colds and other infections. Lavender evaporating at night will aid sleep and promote relaxation.

Specific treatment preparations
These can be blended for special problems such as shingles, chicken pox, mastitis, impetigo, warts and verrucae. The list of problems which can be treated in this way is endless – essences are amazingly versatile!

ESSENTIAL OILS
FROM A-Z

Aniseed
Latin name **Pimpinella anisum**
Oil extracted from the seeds of the plant.
Warning: Aniseed oil can cause irritation to sensitive skins.

Points of interest
Particularly favoured by the Romans, who used the seeds to sweeten breath, as an aphrodisiac, to relieve flatulence and stimulate milk flow. Today it is used to flavour medicines, confectionary and dental preparations. Thought to help alleviate the effects of a hangover!

Special points
Anti-spasmodic and carminative
• A general stimulant, helps relieve flatulence, colic and indigestion.
• Stimulating to the respiratory tract, helpful for asthma, coughs, colds and sore throats.
• Anti-spasmodic effect also helps relieve period pains.
• Galactagogue – useful post-natally to help stimulate milk flow.
• Anti-parasitic – has been proved useful in the treatment of lice and scabies.

NOTE: Aniseed has been avoided by many therapists due to suspected side-effects. The cheap alcoholic drink 'Absinthe' contained alcohol distilled from wormwood, which had a very bitter taste. The aniseed was used to conceal the taste. It was not, however, the cause of the side-effects. It must be emphasized that it was the wormwood which resulted in the highly toxic effects (of brain damage and addiction) not the aniseed.

Bergamot
Latin name **Citrus aurantium sub bergamia**
Obtained by expression from the fruit peel.
Warning: This oil is phototoxic. Do not use before exposure to sun (or sunbed) as the oil may cause pigmentation of the skin.

Aniseed

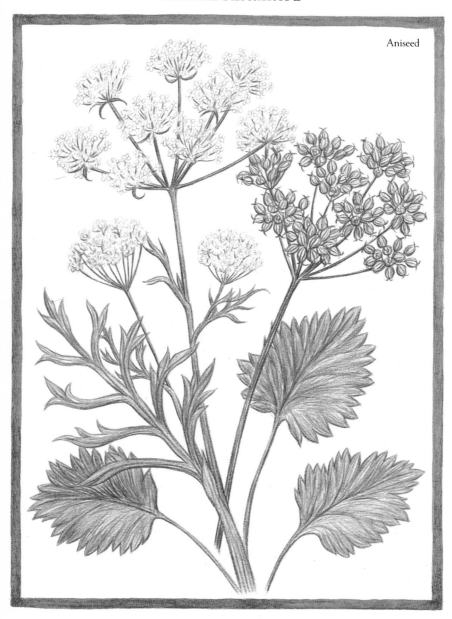

Points of interest
- One of the most versatile and the most popular oils.
- In the past many used the oil to combat intestinal parasites.
- Bergamot is the flavour of Earl Grey tea.

Special points
Helpful for many skin conditions
Antiseptic effect – special affinity for mucous membranes.
Anti-depressant.
- Skin conditions such as eczema, psoriasis, acne and ulcers often respond to bergamot. It is especially indicated where stress and depression are a causative factor in, or the result of, the skin condition. The essence can be used in skin preparations of creams and lotions, and facial oils. Where infection is present, hot compresses are useful to help draw out infection and eliminate toxins (diet and life-style should also be examined).
- Bergamot helps ease the discomfort of chicken pox, shingles and cold sores. It is combined with eucalyptus and added to alcohol or oil and dabbed on eruptions. This also quickens the recovery period.
- Throat and urinary tract infections also respond well to bergamot – in inhalations, gargles or added to baths. Its expectorant effect is particularly helpful for bronchial infections, combined with lemon essence and again used in inhalations.
- Urinary infections such as cystitis, thrush, etc, again respond to bergamot in baths, especially hip baths (sitz).
- Confusion exists between the herb bergamot (*Monarda didyma*) and bergamot oil. The herb is a plant from the New World used as a carminative and remedy for colds. The extractable *thymol* from Monarda is a strong antiseptic with anti-parasitical properties.
- Bergamot oil has been used in cases of piebald skin (vitiligo).

Emotional properties
As an uplifting anti-depressant, bergamot is invaluable for many forms of tension, worry and anxiousness. It is popular with men and women alike. It is also particularly useful for those who tend to binge when feeling at an emotionally low ebb, and seems to help regulate appetite.

Those who are prone to attacks of cystitis and other repeated infections are often suffering from worry or depression. The importance of the holistic approach is underlined here, and the double action of the oils is shown to be particularly useful.

Caraway
Latin name **Carum carvi**
Oil is obtained by distillation of the seeds of the plant. Has a characteristic aroma.

Warning: May cause dermal irritation – use with care.

Points of interest
- The seeds called 'fruits' are a popular herb, used in rye bread, cheeses, liquers and various cakes.
- In European folklore it was believed that caraway would prevent the theft of anything that contained it! It was also included in love potions, given to a lover to prevent them from being 'stolen'.
- It helps eradicate mange in dogs.
- Thought to help those suffering from vertigo.
- It has been fed to pigeons to keep them at home.

Special points
- Used for digestive complaints – a carminative.
- It is indicated as a digestive aid – for gastric spasm, flatulence, stomach distension and indigestion. It is also a galactagogue, thus useful during breast feeding.

Cassia
Latin name **Cinnamonum cassia**
Oil is distilled from leaves and twigs.

Warning: Can cause irritation to sensitive skins.

Points of interest
A very warm spicy smell, similar to cinnamon.
A yellow/brown oil which darkens with age and becomes more viscous.

Special points
- Astringent.
- Tonic.

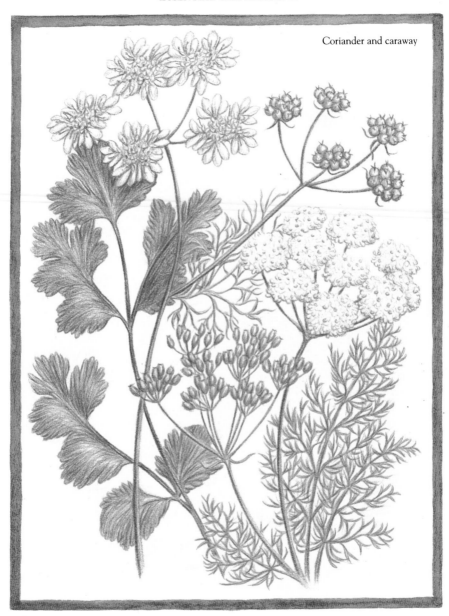

Coriander and caraway

- Used for coughs and colds in inhalations.
- Diarrhoea and stomach ache.
- Headaches.
- Fungicidal, anti-viral, anti-bacterial.
- Hypotensive.

Cedarwood
Latin name **Juniperus virginiana**

Warning: Under no circumstances to be taken internally, nor used during pregnancy. Irritant to sensitive skins.

Points of interest
- One of the first essences to be extracted.
- Used by the Egyptians in their mummification process. The ancients also used it for cosmetics and impregnating papyrus leaves to prevent attack by insects (the wood was also the only one used to make their coffins).
- A good insect repellent.

Special points
Affinity for the respiratory and urinary tracts.
- Cedarwood was used by the north American Indians for respiratory infections where excess catarrh is a specific problem (bronchitis reacts particularly well). Use in inhalation.
- Used for urinary tract infections especially when a painful burning sensation occurs when urinating. It is said to help gonorrhoea and kidney infections too. Use in massage treatments and baths.
- In New Mexico, Indians used cedarwood for skin rashes. Has had some reputation for the treatment of arthritis and rheumatism. For dandruff, a treatment preparation with cedarwood, rosemary and eucalyptus diluted in vegetable oil has an excellent effect.

Chamomile
Latin name **Chamaemelum nobile** formerly *Anthemis nobilis*
(Roman chamomile); *Matricaria recutita* (German chamomile).
Oil distilled from the flowers of the plant.

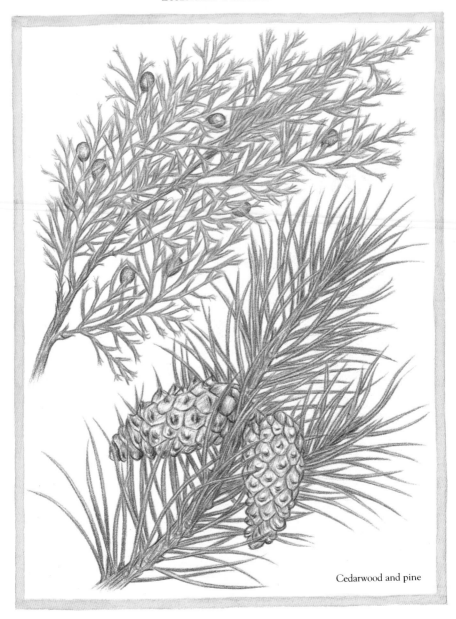

Cedarwood and pine

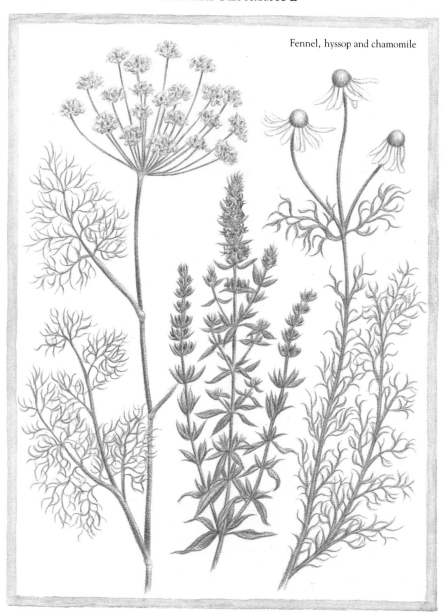

Fennel, hyssop and chamomile

Warning: Chamomile can cause irritation for those with sensitive skins.

Points of interest
Roman chamomile is deep blue in colour due to the high concentration of azulene. Chamomile tea with lactose (milk sugar), if taken after antibiotics, will help restore the normal balance to the intestinal flora.

Special points
- Anti-inflammatory.
- Astringent.
- Cooling febrifuge action.
- Anti-spasmodic.
- Carminative – for flatulence and acute stomach complaints.
- Used for speeding up the healing process of wounds, especially gastric ulcers and has a preventative action taken as herbal tea. Haemorrhoids also respond, as does colitis.
- Chamomile also has an anti-toxic action, is antiseptic and cleansing.
- Inhalations containing chamomile when used for respiratory infections help relieve bacterial toxins.
- Chamomile is beneficial in allergic conditions, probably due to its anti-inflammatory action.
- This oil also stimulates skin cell growth.
- Dysmenorrhoea – use chamomile in baths and massage.
- Particularly useful for mental stress and anxiety and nervous excitability, especially in children.

Cinnamon (bark)
Latin name **Cinnamomum zeylanicum**
Oils distilled from the bark.

Warning: Reports of irritation for those with sensitive skin. Use with care.

Points of interest
- Yellow oil which becomes brown with age.

Special points
- Promotes appetite – useful for sufferers of anorexia.
- Carminative.

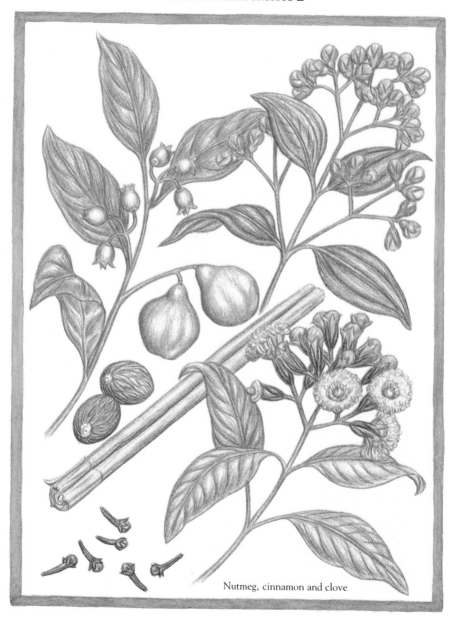

Nutmeg, cinnamon and clove

- Treat colds with inhalations and peppermint for influenza.
- Antiseptic.

Citronella
Latin name **Cymbopogon nardus**
Obtained by distillation from the grass.

Points of interest
- Used by the Chinese for rheumatic pain.
- Fragrance similar to melissa and same action.

Special points
- Use diluted on temples at night in case of sleeplessness.
- Neuralgia.
- Headaches.
- Migraine.
- Insect repellent.

Clove (bud)
Latin name **Eugenia caryophyllus**
Oil is distilled from the dried-flower buds.

Warning: Clove bud oil can produce skin irritation if used neat or in high concentration on sensitive skin.

Points of interest
- Used in many natural-based toothpastes.
- Strong insect repellent, especially useful as a moth repellent.

Special points
- Antispetic (strong).
- Anti-spasmodic.
- Local analgesic used traditionally on cotton wool as toothache 'plug'. Prolonged use can damage the gingival (gum) tissues. Also used for neuralgia.
- Particularly strong antiseptic properties, helpful in cases of diarrhoea and indigestion.
- Anti-spasmodic effect, particularly helpful in asthma and bronchitis.

Eucalyptus
Latin name **Eucalyptus globulus**
Oil extracted from the fresh leaves of the tree.

Warning: Use this very strong essence very sparingly. One or two drops in any blend will be sufficient.

Points of interest
- Aborigines used the strong antiseptic qualities of eucalyptus for injuries to prevent infections and for reducing fevers.
- Eucalyptus is one of the strongest natural antiseptics.
- There are approximately 300 species of eucalyptus but only 15 of these yield good-quality essence.
- Eucalyptus trees were planted in swampy areas to deter mosquitoes. The huge root system helps drain their breeding ground and the insect repellent quality discourages the insects.
- It is one of the largest trees in the world, growing up to 300 feet.

Special points
Strong antiseptic.
Indicated for respiratory problems.
Useful for some skin conditions.
Diuretic.
- The strong anti-viral, bactericidal antiseptic and expectorant action of this essence renders it invaluable for most respiratory infections. Using it in inhalations is particularly effective as it helps kill off the invading microbes as they attack.
- It can be used as an air spray in sick rooms to kill off airborne microbes and freshen the room.
- It is extremely effective in bringing high temperatures down by using cold compresses on the forehead, hands and feet (so effective this has to be monitored carefully; if the temperature is brought down too quickly the person will go into shock).
- It is an effective local pain killer (chicken pox, cold sores, shingles) and also mildly anti-spasmodic. Useful for muscular sprain and discomfort (also indicated for rheumatoid arthritis).
- For urinary tract infections where discharge is present, cystitis, herpes, gonorrhoea (eucalyptus produces an increase in the rate of urea excretion).

Recent research has shown that eucalyptus oil applied as a rub penetrates the lungs. This action has proved extremely useful in the case of respiratory infection.

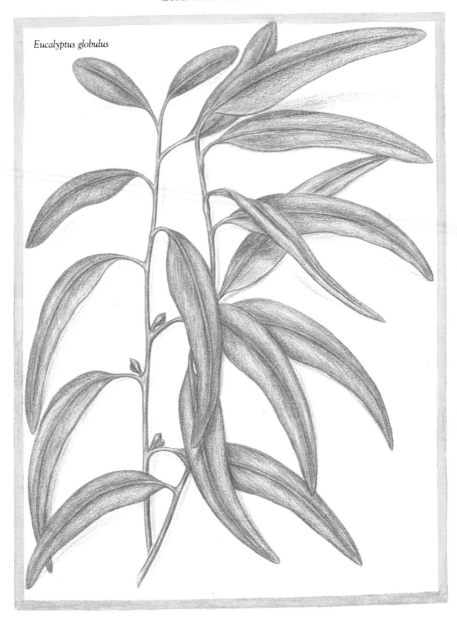

Eucalyptus globulus

Fennel
Latin name **Foeniculum vulgare**
Oil extracted from the seeds of the plant.

Warning: Not to be used on sensitive skin and not to be used before exposure to the sun – phototoxic.

Points of interest
- Roman soldiers chewed fennel seeds during marches when they had no time for a meal.
- Fennel was hung over cottage doors to protect against witchcraft or the evil eye.
- Particularly useful for alcohol poisoning and gout as it helps prevent toxic waste from building up. Thus this oil can play an important role in the treatment and rehabilitation of alcoholics, and has also been used in cases of liver regeneration.

Special points
- Expectorant.
- Diuretic.
- Anti-spasmodic.
- Digestive problems – carminative plus laxative.
- Emmenagogue – slight oestrogen stimulant.
- Galactagogue – stimulates milk flow.
- Useful for menopausal women as their oestrogen levels decrease. Fennel stimulates oestrogen production, helping lessen unpleasant effects.
- Diuretic nature helps in the treatment of gout (combined with juniper).
- Helps alleviate flatulance and constipation (use in abdomen and lower back massage).
- Fennel tea is particularly useful in cases of diarrhoea and colic, safe to use for children.
- Appetite stimulant – may be useful in cases of anorexia nervosa.

Frankincense
Latin name **Boswellia thurifera**
Obtained by invasion of the bark of the tree.

Points of interest
- Used in perfumery for its marvellous fixative properties.
- Offered as a gift to the infant Jesus, because it was then considered to be as precious as gold (as was myrrh).
- The ancient Egyptians used it in their cosmetic facial preparations. (Again their knowledge is demonstrated – as this is another of the rejuvenating essences).

Special points
- Astringent for skin and catarrhal conditions. Cytophylactc (stimulates cell growth) very warming, comforting action.
- Physically this oil is used to help any condition where excess fluid is present. Those who have perpetual colds, bronchitis, respiratory infections, catarrhal conditions in general and asthma. As asthma is a very frightening condition, frankincense's extremely comforting, soothing effect helps calm the panic which exacerbates the shallow breathing. The upper chest and back should be gently massaged.
- Frankincense is a uterine tonic, and is helpful for those suffering from heavy periods. Also useful for pregnant mothers, during labour too, and after the birth.
- Helpful for urinary tract infections such as cystitis – calms the nervous states of those who tend to suffer from these problems.
- Helps heal stubborn wounds.

Emotional properties
Just as this essence is useful for its physically drying effect, it is emotionally indicated for a metaphysically drying effect too: those who tend to gush, who cannot stop talking. It comforts those who find physical contact difficult (a substitute for a hug!) and those who are frightened, nervous or neurotic.

It is also thought to help those who dwell in the past.

Juniper
*Latin name **Juniperus communis***
Oil is distilled from the dried berries.

Warning: To be avoided by pregnant women and those with severe kidney disease.

Points of interest
- Juniper berries are an important ingredient in gin. Juniper is an appetite stimulant, this is why gin and tonic is often used as an aperitif.
- Poorer quality juniper essence is distilled from the branches and leaves as well as from the berries.

Special points
Urinary tract problems, some skin and respiratory problems and gout respond well to the use of this oil. This is an extremely cleansing detoxifier, and should be used for any problems related to poor toxin elimination and uric acid.
- It dramatically relieves urine retention (this often happens in men who have enlarged prostate glands).
- For piles (haemorrhoids) use in aromatic baths and local washes, creams and lotions. Do not use undiluted (you would regret it!).
- Use in baths and massage for scanty or missing periods.
- Weeping eczema, dermatitis and acne may respond well to the use of juniper as it has an astringent detoxifying effect externally.
- Gout is one of the strongest indicated conditions for the use of juniper, this is caused by build-ups of uric acid in the joints.

Emotional properties
The oil has a cleansing effect on the emotional as well as the physical plane. Those dealing with a large number of people daily (doctors, nurses, mothers, aromatherapists) and feel dazed as a result, will find juniper gently stimulates and revitalizes them (it is also thought to be helpful in a crisis).

Lavender
Latin name **Lavandula officinalis,** also **L. angustifolia**
Oil is distilled from the fresh flowers of the plant.

Points of interest
- The most versatile and safest of all oils.
- Lavender comes from the word *lavare* to wash.
- It was extremely popular with the Romans, who probably introduced it to England.
- A strong cytophylactc – a stimulant of cell growth.

Lavender

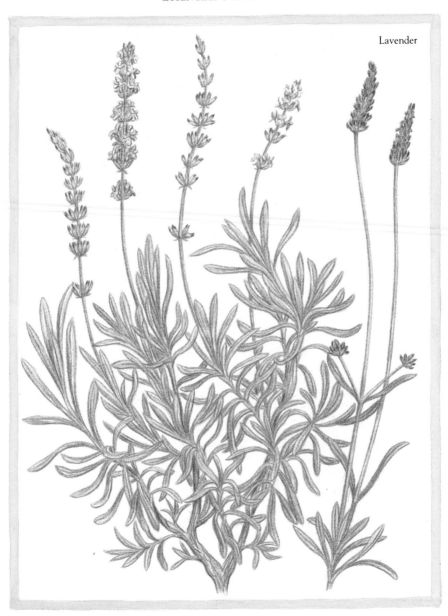

Special points
- Helpful in the treatment of many skin conditions – including burns.
- A general tonic which stimulates bile production.
- Gentle sedative.
- Anti-spasmodic and analgesic.
- Has an antiseptic bactericidal effect and is indicated to soothe and reduce inflammation for eczema, dermatitis, acne, etc. Also reduces scarring.
- Can be applied undiluted to a burn to reduce pain and inflammation, lessen scarring, and promote healing free from infection.
- Very useful for muscular aches and pains, as it soothes and relieves spasm – used in massage.
- Period pains are soothed by using lavender in lower back and abdomen massage. A hot compress of lavender is also very comforting.
- During labour, it helps reduce pain, strengthen contractions and stimulate the expulsion of the afterbirth.
- Lavender is especially useful for children as it has such a gentle action.
- Useful for most infections, especially sinusitis, catarrhal coughs, sore throats. Helps soothe and relieve congestion and attacks bacteria causing the infection.
- The evaporation of the volatile essence is known to stimulate the brain in a particularly beneficial way.
- A general tonic during and after illness.

Emotional properties
- Particularly indicated for those suffering from tension headaches, even migraines. Massage into forehead and temples. It can also be used in a cold compress applied to forehead or back of neck.
- Insomnia – particularly effective sedative action; aiding sleep and helping regulate sleep patterns. Use in bath before retiring. Sprinkle on handkerchief or pillow at night (for children too).
- Generally an emotionally harmonizing oil which helps to balance emotional extremes caused by stress, shock, worry,

impatience. All these states and more can be helped by this gentle, versatile essence.

Lemongrass
Latin name **Cymbopogon citratus,** also **C. flexuosus**
Oil extracted from the grass itself.

Points of interest
- Used traditionally in Indian medicine for hundreds of years.
- Comes from Brazil, Sri Lanka and parts of South Africa.
- Protects animals from fleas and tics.
- Extremely strong odour.

Special points
Action on the nervous system.
- This oil is particularly useful for stress-related conditions such as colitis (combined with neroli).
- Helps ease muscular aches and pains (combined with rosemary) in massage.
- Research in India shows that lemongrass acts as a sedative on the central nervous system.
- A sedating and refreshing deodorant bath preparation (not more than 3 drops pre-diluted).
- Very strong antiseptic and bactericide and anti-fungal effect; useful in treating infections especially feverish conditions.
- General tonic, stimulating effect on the whole system.
- Not an odour particularly liked by many.

Mandarin
Latin name **Citrus reticulata**
Oil comes from the peel of the fruit.
Warning: Possibly phototoxic.

Points of interest
- The name comes from the fruit which was a traditional gift to the Mandarins of China.
- Particularly useful for children's upsets, due to its gentle action and popular odour.

Special points
- General tonic.

- Digestive stimulant.
- Mandarin's action strengthens the liver and stomach and stimulates them (as does grapefruit). It calms intestinal problems and can be combined with grapefruit, orange or neroli for greater effect.
- Particularly useful for those of fragile disposition – the elderly and children.
- Completely safe to use during pregnancy. Helps prevent stretch marks – combined with lavender and neroli (one drop of each in 10ml (¼fl oz/1tbs) almond; 2mls (½tsp) wheatgerm) especially from fifth month of pregnancy onwards.
- For children's tummy upset, massage abdomen in clockwise direction with mandarin's blend. This will soothe, comfort, help expel gas and relieve discomfort.

Neroli/Orange Blossom
Latin name **Citrus aurantium**
Comes from the flowers of the bitter-orange tree.

Points of interest
(My favourite!)
- The oil is thought to have been named after an Italian princess, who discovered the scent.
- It is one of the ingredients of a true eau-de-cologne.
- Orange blossom flowers are traditionally used in bridal bouquets. It is distinctly possible that this is due to the slightly hypnotic effect of this essence!

Special points
One of the strongest stress-relieving oils. It has premarily an emotional effect, although it is indicated for acute stress-related problems, such as:
Colitis.
Palpitations.
Insomnia.
Diarrhoea.
- When chronic diarrhoea is related to stress, shock or nervous tension, neroli will help redress the balance by calming and promoting relaxation. Palpitations and cardiac spasm respond to

Neroli/Orange blossom

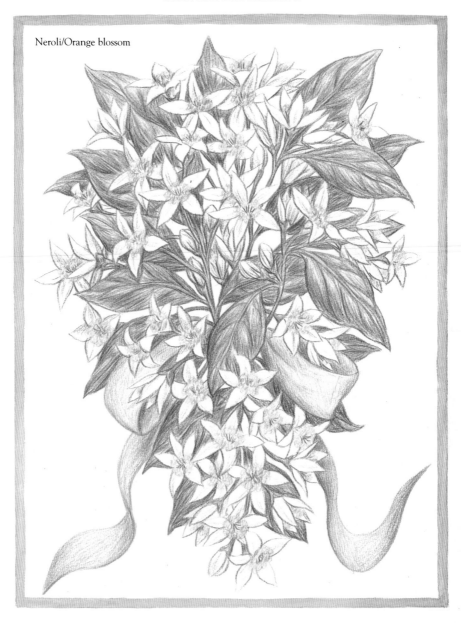

the calming action neroli has on the heart, decreasing the amplitude of the heart muscle contractions. Massage and aromatic baths are the best method of application here, to help alleviate any tension held in the muscles and body posture which need relaxing and re-educating if the person is to truly relax.

• Neroli is one of the skin rejuvenating oils, which is indicated for scarring, thread veins, stretch marks and dry, sensitive skin.

Emotional properties
This special essence is one of the most precious for our stress-related problems: shock, hysteria, sorry fear, nervousness before an exam or interview. Any thoughts that are preventing us from 'switching off', any stress cycle that affects our sleep pattern, our digestion, our energy – neroli is appropriate. It will calm and soothe the body, mind and spirit.

Nutmeg
*Latin name **Myristica fragrans***
Comes from the kernel of the fruit of the tree.

Warning: Do not use over long periods or in high concentrations as this can cause hallucinations and hypnosis. Do not use during pregnancy.

Points of interest
• Trees are male or female and one male can fertilize 20 female trees.
• The trees can grow up to 45ft (14m) high and can produce 1,500 – 2,000 nuts annually, for between 10 to 30 years.

Special points
• Strong stimulant (to be used with carminative to relieve flatulence).
• Stimulates circulation, heartbeat, menstruation (useful in cases of scanty periods), appetite, digestion.
• Used in massage, has an anti-inflammatory action.

A warming oil to be used in the winter, particularly enjoyable when combined with orange.

CAUTION: **Always dilute – even for a bath – for dermal irritation can occur.**

Parsley

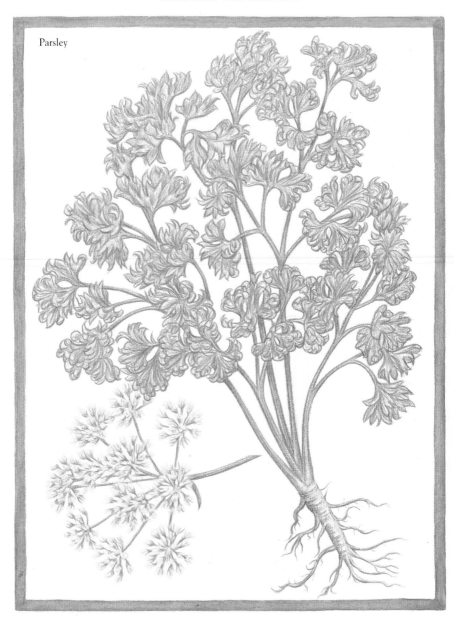

Parsley
Latin name **Petroselinum crispum**
Oil distilled from the seeds.

Warning: Not to be used during pregnancy.

Points of interest
• Although it grows in many temperate climes, it originates from Greece.

Special points
• Emmenagogue (useful in cases of dysmenorrhoea).
• Diuretic.
• Febrifuge – helps bring down temperature.
• Its diuretic properties render it useful for urinary tract infections, and it is said to help break down kidney and bladder stones.
• Parsley is a digestive aid, and so is its essence, which helps ease griping pains of indigestion, and helps expel gas.
• Has a tonic effect on the uterus, and can be used during labour.
• Circulatory tonic too, used in an ointment for piles (anti-inflammatory).
• It is thought to help with liver regeneration.
• Can be useful for asthma.

Patchouli
Latin name **Pogostemon patchouli**
Comes from the leaf of the plant.

Points of interest
• This is one of the very few oils which improves with age.
• Has a cell regenerating action on the skin (also lavender, neroli, tangerine and mandarin).
• It is used in Japan and Malaysia for poisonous snake bites and stings.
• Patchouli has a very unusual hot, oriental, musty odour which is either loved or hated.
• It is thought to be an aphrodisiac.

Patchouli

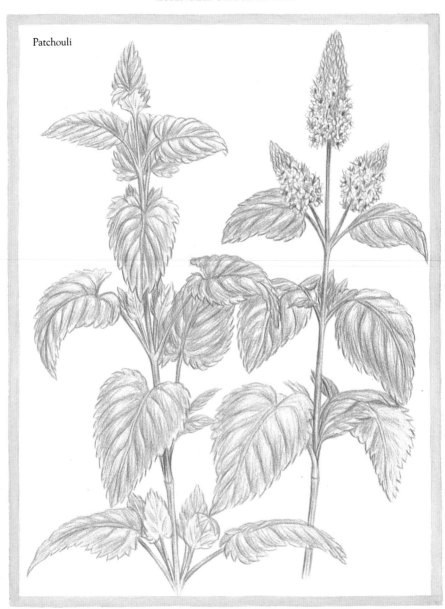

- Insect repellent.

Special points
- Carminative.
- Antiseptic, anti-fungal, anti-bacterial.
- Diuretic.
- Anti-inflammatory.
- Anti-depressant.
- Treatment of skin problems.
- Due to the above properties, the essence is particularly useful in skin preparations for acne and some forms of eczema. It is used when skin is red and sore from an allergic reaction.
- As it is anti-fungal, athlete's foot can be treated, as can dandruff (when combined with cedarwood and rosemary).
- With its skin regenerating action it is particularly indicated for scar tissue, cracked skin and the more mature skin type.

Emotional properties
For those who like the smell, this oil can have a strong anti-depressant action. It is also said to be an aphrodisiac.

Peppermint
Latin name **Mentha piperita**

Warning: Not to be used by pregnant women. To be used generally in very small quantities (1 drop per blend). Can be irritating to the skin. Not to be used by those with sensitive skin.

Points of interest
- There are 25 species of mints and hundreds of hybrids; it is one of the most used essences today. Used in the manufacture of medicines, confectionary, liquors, deodorants, toothpastes and cigarettes.
- Due to its strong odour, it was scattered on the floors of houses and in public places, to mask foul odours and repel insects, rats and mice.
- Mint leaves make a delicious and beneficial addition to any salad.
- Very strong antiseptic properties.

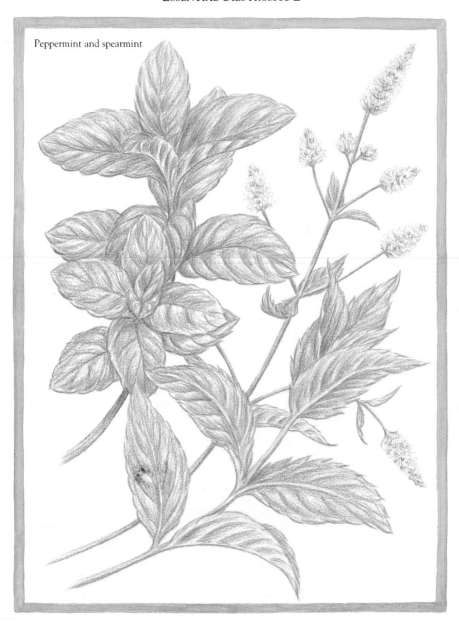

Peppermint and spearmint

Special points
- Care should be taken when using peppermint essence since even the vapours can cause irritation to the eyes.
- Not to be used if homoeopathic remedies are being taken.
- Do not use in the evening as the strongly stimulating effect will keep you awake.
- Classic digestive remedy.
- Anti-spasmodic.
- Digestive and general stimulant.
- The analgesic, cooling effect can help alleviate headaches, even migraines, in a cold compress or inhalation (sniffing a drop on a tissue).
- Travel sickness, especially in children can be alleviated by a sniff of peppermint on a tissue.
- Digestive problems such as indigestion, stomach pains, flatulance, irritable bowel syndrome, can all be relieved by a gentle abdominal massage with a drop of peppermint in the base oil.
- Nausea and vomiting through shock often respond to inhaling a drop or two of peppermint. If the sickness is due to an infection the peppermint will also help due to its strong antiseptic qualities. Peppermint tea is also indicated in association with such problems.
- Respiratory disorders respond well to a drop of peppermint in an inhalation due to its anti-inflammatory effect. Sinus headaches and migraine headaches will also respond to a compress with one drop of peppermint.
- A compress will also help relieve mastitis and cool down feverish patients (compress on hands and feet).
- As a stimulant, it is useful when mental clarity is required, it 'clears the head'.
- Emotionally it is useful for shock, hysteria, paralysis and palpitations through shock.
- One drop can be added to inhalations for bronchitis and colds to help relieve congestion. (Remember to close your eyes when inhaling).
- Dysmenorrhoea.
- Anti-rheumatic.

Petitgrain
Latin name **Citrus bigardia**
Oil distilled from the leaves and twigs.

Points of interest
- Name originates from the tiny unripe oranges – the size of cherries looking like 'little grains' from which the essence used to be distilled.
- Used extensively in the perfume industry.

Special points
- Can be used as an inexpensive substitute for neroli (in serious cases of anxiety, depression or insomnia the real thing should be used).
- Has good deodorant qualities and makes a refreshing aromatic bath.
- Can be used in a final hair rinse to impart a lovely scent.

Pine
Latin name **Pinus sylvestris**
Oil distilled from the needles, young twigs and cones.

Warning: Make sure that the oil you are using has the Latin name above, as other species may be hazardous.

Points of interest
- North American Indians used extract of pine needles to prevent scurvy.
- In North America the needles were also made into mattress stuffing, 'pine wool', which reputedly warded off lice and fleas.

Special points
- Strong antiseptic.
- Strong expectorant/decongestant.
- Circulation stimulant.
- Particularly indicated in inhalations for respiratory conditions with excess catarrh:
Bronchitis
Sinusitis

Sore throats
Flu
Pneumonia.

Always seek advice from a general practitioner if the condition is serious.

- Very effective when used in conjunction with eucalyptus and tea-tree.
- Has antiseptic properties as it is also a digestive stimulant and helps soothe intestinal pains and gas.
- A circulation stimulant also indicated for:
Arthritis, rheumatism
Neuralgia and nervous diseases
Gout
Muscular pains.

A hot pine bath is useful in cases of rheumatism, neuralgia and nervous diseases. A rest after a hot bath is beneficial.

Rose Geranium
Latin name **Pelargonium graveolens**
Oil is distilled from the leaves and flowers of the plant.

Warning: Can cause irritation to sensitive skins.

Points of interest
- Geranium is an insect repellent, perhaps this is the reason they are popular in window boxes!
- Very antiseptic and haemostatic (helps stop bleeding) thus it is a useful oil to use in the treatment of injuries.
- Used in many skin preparations due to its antiseptic nature.
- This oil stimulates the adrenal cortex, the hormones secreted by this area are basically regulators. Geranium therefore, helps to regulate hormonal imbalances.

Special points
- A very harmonizing effect.
- Useful for skin conditions.
- In my experience geranium is extremely useful in treating all

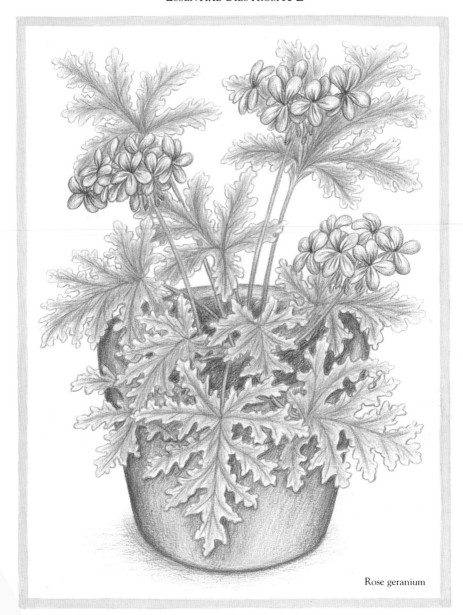

Rose geranium

hormone related disorders (very female essence) helps with menopausal problems, hot flushes, etc.
- Pre-menstrual tension (PMT) responds well, as does water retention at this time, as the oil has a diuretic effect too.
- Cellulitis and mastitis also benefit from the use of this oil, combined with massage work on lymphatic drainage points (and drinking plenty of mineral water!) due to its astringent nature.
- The geranium's mildly analgesic and sedative qualities also have a good effect on diarrhoea and peptic ulcers.
- Serious skin conditions, such as eczema, burns, shingles, ringworm and lice, all respond to this amazing oil – due to its anti-fungal and antiseptic properties.

Emotional properties
This is an oil particularly indicated for emotional extremes – those who are up one minute and down the next. This state often coincides with a change in hormone levels, so yet again the oil can be seen to work on different levels to achieve the desired effect.

Geranium is also very cleansing, and as with other flower oils, is very useful for those with nervous problems and anxiety.

Rosemary
Latin name **Rosmarinus officinalis**
The oil is distilled from the leaves of the plant.

Warning: To be avoided during pregnancy.

Points of interest
- The herb is used in cooking not only due to its taste but because it has a preserving nature.
- When used as a muscular rub for long-distance runners, it helps prevent muscular strain.
- An ingredient in traditional eau-de-cologne.

Special points
- Emmenagogue.
- Anti-bacterial and anti-oxidant.
- Strong stimulant, analgesic and tonic.
- Used for headaches, neuralgia and sciatica.

Rosemary

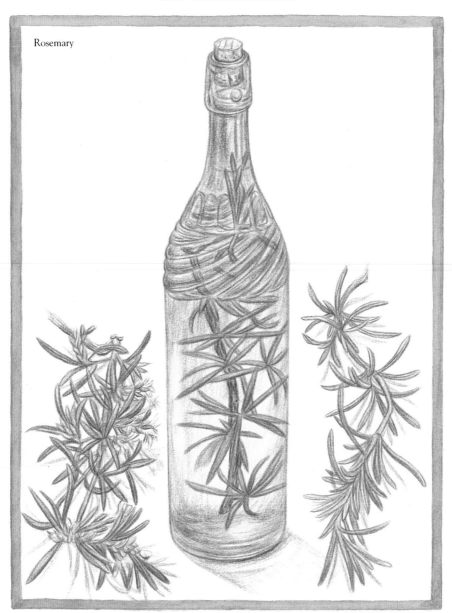

- Used for poor circulation – acts as a counter irritant and speeds up circulation and removal of toxins. Therefore indicated for:
Varicose veins
Arthritis (unless very hot and inflammed)
Muscular aches and sprains (analgesic effect and anti-inflammatory)
- Stimulating morning bath for those with poor circulation, tension or hypotension – has a general tonic effect.
- Inhalation for respiratory problems, catarrh, flu, colds and sinusitis.
- Useful for digestive problems, flatulence, stomach pains, constipation. Has a stimulating anti-spasmodic action, and a tonic effect on the stomach.
- For skin and hair care. Brings a shine to dark hair when used as a rinse. Helps thinning hair when used regularly as it stimulates blood supply to hair follicles (especially helpful if hair loss is due to illness).
- Promotes perspiration.
- Dandruff – when used in treatment for this candida infection, it helps kill the candida.
- Makes an astringent tonic for oily skin.
- Refreshing bath for exhaustion, not to be used before bed due to its stimulating effect.

Emotional properties
- Indicated for the sluggish and apathetic. Has a strong stimulant effect on the mind, clearing the head and clarifying thoughts. Can have an uplifting, anti-depressant effect.

Sage
Latin name *Salvia officinalis*
Oil distilled from the whole herb.

Warning: Not to be used during pregnancy.

Points of interest
- Helps to prevent sweating.
- Salvia is from the Latin *salvere* meaning to heal.
- Anti-inflammatory.

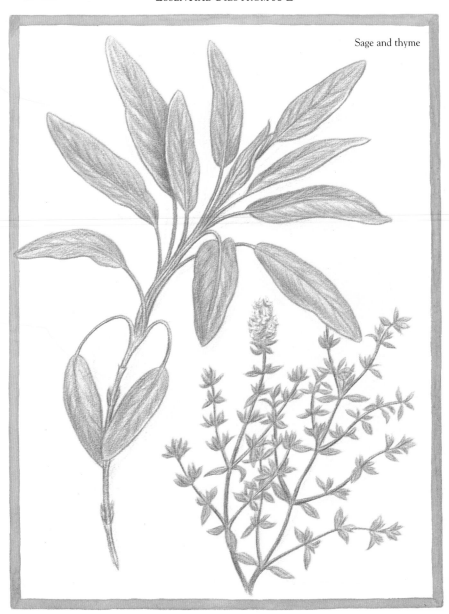

Sage and thyme

- Specific stimulating action on the nervous system.
- Helps relieve period pains and menopausal problems.
- Astringent and cicatrizing (promotes formation of scar tissue) effect, which makes it useful in the general treatment of wounds.
- A useful 'mouth' remedy for:

Sore throats	Antiseptic
Oral thrush	gargle and
Gingivitus	mouthwash
Laryngitis.	DO NOT SWALLOW.

- Blends well with rosemary for nervous disability.

'The said decoction made in wine taketh away the itching of the cods if they be bathed therewith.' Culpeper.

Sandalwood
Latin name **Santalum album**
Distilled from small drips and raspings of the tree's heart wood.

Points of interest
- Has been used for thousands of years in India for both cosmetic and medicinal uses, religious incense and embalming.
- Sandalwood is a parasitic tree which buries its roots in other trees.
- Indian medicine believes it has a beneficial effect on the memory.

Special points
- Strong effect on the genito/urinary system.
- Diuretic.
- Anti-spasmodic.
- Stimulant.
- Respiratory infections.
- Expectorant.
- Sandalwood has a strong antiseptic action on the bladder and kidneys. It is useful for cystitis and other urinary infections, and gonorrhoea (although medical advice must be sought).
- Bronchitis, laryngitis and other catarrhal conditions respond very well to the soothing, antiseptic action. Can be applied to the throat and massaged into the chest and back. Inhalations also appropriate.

- Has a very soothing action on dry, sore or inflammed skin. Also for very oily skin, acne and scabies. Warm compresses can relieve irritation for shaving rashes.
- Astringent effect for diarrhoea.

Emotional properties
Just as sandalwood has a strengthening effect on weak or lost voices, it also gives strength to the emotionally weak and fearful – those who lack self confidence. It is also said to have aphrodisiac properties, perhaps due to its effect on boosting confidence.

Spearmint
Latin name **Mentha spicata/Mentha cariaca**
Oil distilled from the fresh flowers of the plant.

Warning: Can cause irritation of sensitive skins.

Points of interest
- Spearmint taste is less harsh than peppermint, and it is an important commodity in the food industry. It is used to flavour food, liqueurs and teas. Popular flavour with children.
- The United States grows approximately 28,000 acres of spearmint annually.

Special points
- Carminative – helps relieve gas pains.
- A general digestive aid.

Tangerine
Latin name **Citrus nobilis**
Oil expressed from the peel of the fruit.

Warning: Not to be used before exposure to sun – possibly phototoxic.

Points of interest
- This essence is used in conjunction with lemon and orange to accentuate their properties.

Special points
- Aids digestion (stomachic).

- Laxative.
- A tonic for the peripheral circulatory system. Useful to help prevent stretch marks – treats the skin with vitamin C.

Tea-tree/Ti-tree
Latin name **Melaleuca alternifolia**
The oil is distilled from the leaves of the plant.

Points of interest
- Tea-tree contains four substances that do not occur anywhere else in nature.
- Next to thyme it is the most antiseptic of all oils. It is safer to use, and unlike thyme, can be used undiluted (to great effect).
- The presence of infection increases the effectiveness of the action of tea-tree.
- It is currently being used in trials on a number of different conditions, including Aids, with promising results.
- It is used in Australia extensively. Dentists use tea-tree for mouthwashes, sterilizing cavities before filling, and gum disease. A 4% dilution is used in toothpastes and soaps.

Special points
- Strong disinfectant (stronger than many chemicals).
- Anti-viral.
- Anti-fungal.
- Anti-bacterial.
- Antiseptic.
- Very efficacious in the treatment of urinary tract disorders (in pessaries, douches, sitz baths and on tampons).
- For trichomonal vaginitis, thrush, cystitis and other such infections.
- For respiratory infections – use tea-tree in inhalations, massage, gargles and chest rubs.
- Anti-fungal action works well on athlete's foot, ringworm, warts, verrucae, corns, abscesses. Use in a cream or 5% vegetable oil, or applied neat.
- Also effective and soothing on cold sores. Applied diluted in vegetable oil at 5%.
- Use gargle for mouth ulcers, toothache, bad gums (dental

caries), bad breath, tonsilitis (10 drops in glass of water).
- Soothes and promotes healing for facial spots (undiluted), burns and sunburn (in a cream).
- Lice also respond well! (see page 85).

Thyme
Latin name **Thymus vulgaris**
Oil distilled from the flowers of the plant.

Warning: Never use neat thyme oil on skin. Do not use during pregnancy. Dilute before adding to bath. Do not use on children's skin.

Points of interest
- This oil is distilled twice to remove irritating substances present in the plant itself.
- When used in cooking, it delays the putrification of meat and acts as a digestive aid.
- A much stronger antiseptic than many of its chemical counterparts, or any other essential oil.

Special points
- Anti-spasmodic.
- Most antiseptic essence.
- Expectorant.
- Emmenagogue.
- Diuretic.
- Carminative (aids digestion and expulsion of gas).
- Especially useful for respiratory infections – used in inhalations and mouth gargles (not to be swallowed) in very small dilutions.
- Colds, convulsive coughing, whooping cough.
- Coughs, asthma.
- Any mouth, throat or chest infection.
- Especially indicated for convalescents.
- Stimulates appetite and sluggish digestion.
- Stimulates immune system.
- Central nervous system stimulant.
- Depression is an aftermath of illness which responds well to thyme.

- Diuretic action helps arthritis, gout, muscular aches and sprains, as it speeds up circulation and aids the removal of uric acid.
- Stimulates absent or scanty menstruation.
- For boils and sores and other infected skin problems.
- Deodorant.

Emotional properties
Thyme has an uplifting effect on depressive, apathetic states, nervous anxiety and exhaustion. It assists insomniacs too.

West Indian Bay
Latin name **Myrcia acris**
Oil is extracted from the leaves of the plant.

Points of interest
It was used as the hair tonic 'Bay Rum' in previous times.

Special points
- Astringent.
- Antiseptic, decongestant, tonic.
- Used to treat respiratory conditions and colds.

Ylang Ylang
Latin name **Cananga odorata**
Comes from the flowers.

Points of interest
- Used in the popular Victorian 'macassar oil', due to the tonic effect Ylang has on the scalp.
- The flowers are pink, mauve and yellow. The best oil comes from the yellow flowers.
- Native name 'Ylang Ylang' means flower of flowers.

Special points
- Tachycardia (fast pulse), aphrodisiac.
- Palpitations.
- Hyperpnoea (rapid breathing).
- High blood-pressure (which often accompanies one or more of the above).

Ylang ylang

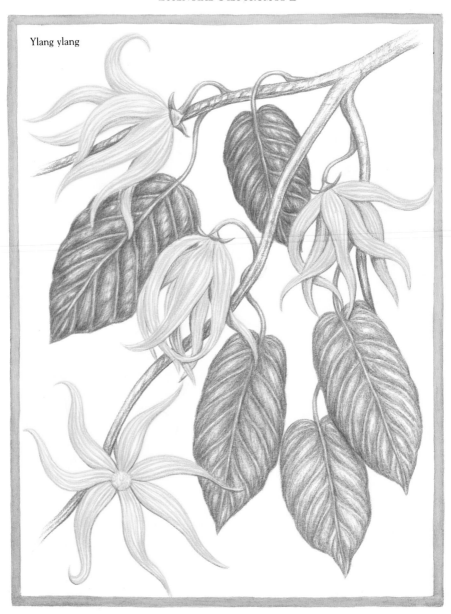

• Ylang helps slow down rapid breathing, abnormally rapid heart beat and irregular heart beat, when due to stress.
• For sexual problems, Ylang is very helpful on the emotional and physical plane. It has a soothing, relaxing, anti-depressant effect. This will help calm and soothe the anxious, impatient states which may lead to, or be attributed to, sexual problems.

Vetiver
Latin name **Vetiveria zizanioides**
Oil is extracted from the roots of the wild grass.

Points of interest
• The oil is called 'The Oil of Tranquillity' where it is cultivated, in India and Sri Lanka.
• Used as a fixative in perfumery.

Special properties
• Extremely calming, used to treat anxiety and nervous tension.

Massage

WHEN TO AVOID MASSAGE

Always check with your medical practitioner before giving a massage to anyone suffering from serious illness. Do not massage in the following cases (unless specifically advised by your doctor):

- Severe heart disease.
- Epilepsy.
- Fever.
- Recent fracture.
- Recent scar tissue.
- Severe bruising.
- Haemorrhage. (Do not massage those with a medical history of haemorrhaging. You could, by stimulating the circulation, cause a blood clot to travel which could be dangerous.)
- Acute inflammation.
- Areas contaminated by contagious skin disease.
- Septic areas (application of essential oil such as tea-tree may be enormously beneficial).
- Very bad sunburn.
- Very high or very low blood-pressure.
- Coronary.
- Recently diagnosed diabetes (only massage diabetics if the correct insulin balance has been obtained. Use gentle treatment, and keep the diabetic warm, as they are insensitive to temperature changes. Pay particular attention after the massage, and bring the person around slowly).
- Avoid pressure over the abdomen during menstruation (heavy pressure could increase flow).
- Avoid pressure over abdomen during pregnancy.
- After a heavy meal.
- Varicose veins (massage in the early stages can help prevent these. Pressure over a large varicose vein may rupture the weakened vein wall).
- Open wounds.
- Nausea.
- A bacterial/viral infection, such as pneumonia. (As the blood

and lymph circulation is stimulated, the temperature may be raised, and the infection spread. Massage may help during the recuperation period.)
- Areas of unrecognized lumps (**seek medical advice**).

DIFFERENT FORMS OF MASSAGE

Massage is, by its very nature, incredibly versatile. It stimulates the blood and lymphatic circulation, relieves muscular tension, stimulates the release of body chemicals, passively exercises and re-educates the muscles, aids desquamation (shedding of dead skin cells) – the list is endless.

Just as the list of massage properties is almost endless, so is the different forms of massage. The strength, direction, and application of pressure varies according to the method involved. No one form of treatment supersedes another. Many aromatherapists use a combination of methods within each treatment.

These are some of the most popular methods used both as a form of treatment in their own right, and incorporated into aromatherapy treatments.

Swedish massage

Swedish massage, otherwise known as the 'Ling System', was developed by Per Henrik Ling in the early nineteenth century. He split up some of the ancient massage movements into specific techniques, analyzed them, and explained why they were used. This is one of the most basic forms of massage from which many others subsequently developed. It is a fairly superficial but none the less valuable method, which is practised today by many beauty therapists. It consists of an 'all over' body massage, designed to assist blood circulation, lymphatic drainage and to manipulate the soft tissues. The effect is pleasantly relaxing.

Remedial massage

This is a more specialized form of massage treatment used for muscular problems and injury. Deep tissue work is applied to stimulate circulation, release muscular spasm, soften previously injured and consequently restrictive tissues, sometimes causing discomfort. This is not used primarily to promote relaxation but to treat specific problems.

Mechanical massage

There are two principal types of mechanical massage applicators:
1 Percussors.
2 Gyrators.

1 Percussors are usually small hand-held mechanisms which have a vibratory effect on soft tissue areas. These also include the vibratory belts and chairs used to break down cellulite and exercise the muscles in beauty salons.

2 Gyrators are hand held or upright machines, which are used to mimic the action of the human hand. They are widely used to save the time and energy involved in a massage given by the human hand.

Essential oils are often not to be used with these machines as they corrode the rubber or plastic heads.

Shiatsu

This is an ancient eastern form of massage involving pressure application with the fingers, thumbs, elbows, knees and even the feet! This works on the principle that when the natural energy flow of the system becomes upset, symptoms of disease are the result. The energies within our bodies flow along invisible lines or meridians. Shiatsu pressure along certain points on these lines ('tsubos') restores the weakened or blocked flow. A point which is blocked is usually sensitive or painful, and there is often a small indentation where a point is located. Regular shiatsu treatment therefore offers powerful preventative treatment. There are about 600 shiatsu points throughout the body. Some basic points can be useful for treatment in the home.

NOTE: Acupressure is a similar technique using finger pressure *only* to balance the energy flow.

Reflexology

What is it and how does it work?

This is another ancient and fascinating healing art, dating back thousands of years. The ancient Egyptians used reflexology, which is shown on beautiful paintings found in the pyramids.

Reflexology works on the principle that there are different zones or reflex points in the hands and feet, which correspond to different glands, organs and areas in the body. A professionally trained reflexologist can ascertain various weaknesses or disorders about which even the subject is sometimes unaware. Where a congested area exists, the area is usually tender when pressure is applied. Tiny crystalline deposits can be detected under the surface of the skin. Pressure applied to these areas helps to stabilize the system by clearing the congestion.

The main benefits
1 Reflexology is a very effective way of alleviating stress and its many different actions on the body.
2 A form of reflexology can be used in conjunction with massage and other therapies to complement each other.
3 The immune system derives particular benefit from the decongestant action on the lymph and endocrine glands.
4 The general balance and well-being of the system (homeoestasis) greatly benefits from the boost to the circulatory system.
5 Once instructed a subject can continue to work on the relevant points, on a 'self-help' basis.
6 Reflexology, in common with all true Natural Health Therapies, works on a completely holistic basis, taking the whole person into consideration.

NOTE: It must be underlined that a reflexologist should never diagnose a specific complaint, as messages can be conflicting. This should not, however, deflect from the overall benefits that this therapy offers.

BEFORE YOU START
How the oils are chosen
By a professional aromatherapist
A holistic aromatherapist will decide which essential (and base oils) to use during a lengthy consultation process. This will take into consideration the subject's medical history, stress levels, dietary habits, exercise routine, any complaints, and general emotional thoughts and feelings. An accurate individual assessment is then formed and certain essential oils chosen; advice is given, following the consultation.

At home

Using aromatherapy in the home is not quite as involved. Certain information should be obtained, however, to help choose the right essence, or blend of essences, for each person. It is likely that your subject is a close friend or relative. You will probably know how the person is feeling, but it is important not to assume this. They may not have mentioned that they have recently been sleeping badly, or have a persistent headache, for instance.

Ask your subject if they have any specific complaints. Ascertain whether their medical history includes anything out of the ordinary. **Check the list of contra-indications before proceeding.** Try and pick up on any messages their body or facial expression may show, such as hunched round shoulders, restricted neck movement or a furrowed brow. Consider their emotional state. Are they generally nervous, tense people who need relaxing with oils such as lavender, chamomile or clary sage? Or are they in need of a generally stimulating treatment with oils such as rosemary, eucalyptus or thyme? Cold hands and feet, cellulite and muscular tension will all indicate the use of certain essences.

Remember to wait at least an hour after a meal before you give or receive a massage. This will enable your body to digest the food properly, preventing indigestion or the necessity of avoiding abdominal massage.

You

There are a few basic points to remember before you give a massage.

● Ensure you have read the list of contra indications in this chapter before proceeding.

● Hands should be clean.

● Nails should be short (so that you do not scratch your subject!).

● Wear loose comfortable washable clothing.

● Be aware of your posture. Keep your back straight at all times. This applies whether your subject is on a couch or on the floor. (It is easy to strain the back, and then you will be the one who needs treatment!)

- Do not apply deep pressure unless qualified to do so.
- Do not work on any area that is very painful. Consult a medically qualified practitioner if you are in doubt.
- Keep tissues or a cloth handy in case you spill your oil, which should be kept within easy reach during your massage.
- Warm your hands before you begin the massage.
- Do not give treatment if you are felling unwell.

Your subject
- It is advisable for your subject to bath or shower before massage, if possible, the pores of the skin are then dilated, and the essences will be readily absorbed. Cleanliness is also maintained.
- Your subject should be extremely comfortable, or complete relaxation will not occur.
- They must be adequately covered with towels, to maintain warmth and prevent embarrassment.
- If hair is long, pin it back off the neck.

The environment
- It should be warm enough for your partially clad subject to feel comfortable. This is usually a little too hot for the masseur, who is undergoing exercise.
- The light should be adjusted so the subject is not dazzled and the atmosphere is relaxing.
- The telephone should be taken off the hook, to prevent interruption. Soothing music can be played, or peace and quiet maintained – according to preference.
- Evaporating essences in the room add to the aesthetic and therapeutic effect

The massage surface
A professional massage couch obviously provides the optimum surface. These can also be constructed quite easily. The height is important, and should reach the palm of your hand when your arms are by your sides. This helps minimize the likelihood of back strain when giving a massage, and enables the correct pressure to be applied. A head hole in the couch is an excellent addition. This ensures the spine is straight when the subject is lying on

their front. It also prevents neck strain, which may happen if the subject has to rest their head on one side for any length of time.

The floor is also an ideal surface when adequately padded. Using a bed or very soft surface is not recommended. This 'gives' when any pressure is applied, and the subject then derives less benefit. It is also difficult to maintain the correct posture from the masseur's point of view.

Place a duvet, blankets or towels on the floor. Pad adequately with pillows or cushions. These may be placed under the knees and head when your subject is lying on their back. Support the small of the back by placing them under the abdomen, ankles and possibly under the chest. Do not proceed until the subject is completely comfortable and at ease.

The massage
Before you begin, relax and empty your mind of negative thoughts. You may pass these on to your subject. Relax him or her by asking questions during the preliminary analysis. Explain what the massage procedure will entail. Generally, put them at their ease.

You do not need to have professional training to give a good massage. Once you have mastered a few basic techniques you can bring great relief and enjoyment. Do not be afraid of reacting to your intuition.

If time is limited concentrate on one or two areas of the body. The whole system can benefit from a foot massage. The back is generally an area that holds a lot of tension, and it is also a large surface area for the absorption of the oils.

If you are giving someone a massage for the first time, or if your subject is nervous or embarrassed, begin by concentrating on the hands or feet. He or she can then watch, and talk easily, with eye contact. There can be a surprising amount of tension in these areas. During the treatment, watch the person's face, as this will tell you if the area is tender, among other things. Ask your subject to tell you if they particularly like or dislike any movement. They will probably volunteer this information spontaneously.

Be prepared for a form of emotional release. It is an excellent and rewarding sign, as this shows the person is 'letting go'. Most people will just sigh deeply, and this is the point at which you know they have relaxed. Others, particularly those under pressure, or upset, worried or angry, may laugh, cry or talk incessantly. Whatever their reaction, your response should be positive and reassuring. If they seem embarrassed or uneasy at this point, offer congratulations. Explain that when bodily tension is released, negative emotion may also come to the surface.

Having established contact with your subject, do not break that contact until the treatment is finished. This is important, as it is reassuring. Your subject knows where you are even when his or her eyes are closed. It also ensures that you do not make them jump, or wake them up, when you re-establish contact. Pour the oil into the palm of your hand, not straight on to the body. Use a little at a time. Only talk during the massage if your subject wishes to converse. If they are quiet, maintain silence, and let them sleep, think or relax in peace.

ILLUSTRATED GUIDE TO SOME BASIC MASSAGE TECHNIQUES

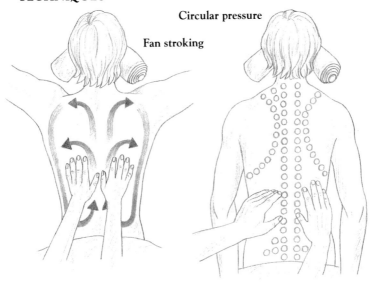

Circular pressure

Fan stroking

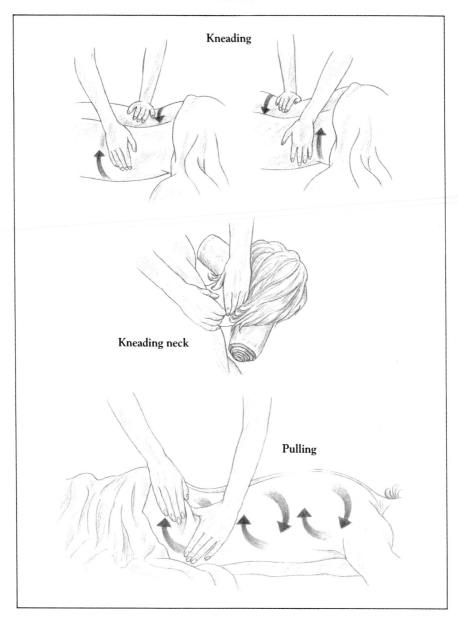

Kneading

Kneading neck

Pulling

GENERAL AILMENTS

GENERAL AILMENTS

The following recommendations are for **adult use**. The different methods of applications come under these basic headings:

Massage oil
2½% dilution (10 drops of essence in 20ml/½fl oz/2 tbs of vegetable oil) unless otherwise directed.

Inhalation
5–10 drops of essence in a bowl of steaming water from which the vapours are then inhaled. Cover bowl and head with towel and inhale with the eyes closed to prevent irritation.

Compress
1–2 drops of essential oil in a bowl of cold, tepid or hot water, according to the treatment advised. A handkerchief or piece of material should be placed gently on the surface of the water to pick up the film of essential oil. Apply accordingly.

Facial preparations
A 1% dilution (5 drops of essence in 20ml/½fl oz/2 tbs of oil, cream or lotion) unless otherwise directed.

Air spray for room freshening
A 2½% dilution – 25 drops of essence in 50ml/2fl oz/¼ cup of water.

Air spray for antiseptic fumigating purposes
A 5% dilution can be sprayed at regular intervals throughout the sickroom. This will freshen the room and reduce the likelihood of the spread of infection. The patient will also benefit from the inhalation of the oils used.

Aromatic baths
5–10 drops of essence diluted in 1–2 tsp of vegetable oil or full fat milk. Agitate the water before use to disperse the droplets.

Sitz baths
5 drops of essence should be added to 1¾l (3pt) of water which should then be sat in to reach the affected area. (This is useful for genito-urinary infections.) Dilute oil in 1tsp (5ml) of vegetable oil, and agitate the water.

GENERAL AILMENTS

Ailment: **Arthritis**

Treatment: Essences used in baths, massage and specific application (osteo-arthritis) are indicated. Rosemary, coriander, lemon, juniper and cypress. Eucalyptus, yarrow and chamomile, clary sage, marjoram and lavender. Use anti-inflammatory oils in cold compress especially after massage treatment, and during a 'flare up'. (Massage should be avoided at this time.) Peppermint can help cool inflammed joints. Dietary supplements also advised; green lipped mussel extract (if no sea food allergy) silica, celery seed, etc

Dilution: Massage oil 2½%–5%. Ointment for specific application 5%.

Baths – 10 drops of essence in 2 tsp (7ml/¼fl oz) vegetable oil. 1 drop of essence per compress

Effect: In baths and massage aim to promote the removal of the excess acid in the joints. Specified ointments speed up circulation and toxin release. Anti-inflammatory oils soothe inflammation and the anti-spasmodic analgesic action helps ease pain and promote movement. Food allergy will exacerbate condition as will lack of exercise, etc. Silica will help break down calcium deposits causing joint deformity

Ailment: **Asthma**

Treatment: Regular aromatherapy treatment can help reduce stress which often triggers attacks. Inhale drops of anti-spasmodic essences such as lavender, marjoram, frankincense, clary sage and neroli from tissue. Chamomile should be used if an allergy triggers an attack. Massage the back to help calm and relieve spasm, and use gentle pressure on shiatsu point lung 1

Dilution: Inhale 2 drops essence neat on tissue. Use 2½% in massage

Effect: These oils help relieve the spasm in the bronchial tubes in the lung. The calming effect helps alleviate panic, and aid deeper breathing (frankincense)

Ailment: **Athlete's foot (and ringworm)**

Treatment: Tea-tree essence, myrrh and lavender indicated. Keep foot **dry**, clean, wear cotton socks and bare feet as much as possible

Dilution: Tea-tree undiluted. Ointment for dry cracked skin (see recipe section)

Effect: Tea-tree and myrrh have an anti-fungal action which kills the mould

Ailment: **Bronchitis**

Treatment: **Acute:** Inhalation (10 drops) 3 times daily. Avoid dairy products which increase mucus formation. (Refined sugar also.) **No smoking**. A short (24-hr) fast may speed up recovery. **Chronic:** Inhalation morning and evening massage may help. Dietary advice, supplements and exercise/life-style should also be considered for both forms of bronchitis. Detoxifying essences indicated for both forms in baths and massage: cedar-wood, juniper and frankincense

Dilution: **Acute** – 3 drops tea-tree; 1 drop eucalyptus; 4 drops lemon; 1 drop peppermint; 1 drop sage

Chronic – 4 drops cedarwood; 3 drops eucalyptus; 3 drops rosemary

Effect: In **Acute** cases this blend of essences will act as a decongestant, loosening mucus. Expectorant, anti-viral, anti-bacterial action also

Massage may help loosen the tightness in the upper thoracic area for **Chronic** sufferers. The inhalations and expectorant action will help get rid of excess phelgm

Ailment: **Bruises**

Treatment: Lavender essence can be applied immediately. Fennel and hyssop are also useful, and an ice-cold compress should be applied to the area as soon as possible. (The homoeopathic remedy arnica is also highly recommended)

Dilution: Undiluted 1 drop of each in cold compress

Effect: Strong analgesic and anti-flammatory action

Ailment: **Burns**
Treatment: For minor burns, apply a few drops of lavender essence to area. For major burns, soak sterile gauze in lavender and apply. Renew every 2 hours. Seek medical advice if burn is severe
Dilution: Undiluted
Effect: Will prevent blistering, infection, reduce pain and likelihood of scarring

Ailment: **Cellulite**
Treatment: Drink at least a pint of pure (mineral, distilled or reverse osmosis) water daily. Exercise and massage using essential oils have an excellent effect. Aromatic baths also indicated. (Diet and life-style must be analyzed.) Essences include rosemary, cypress, geranium, juniper and fennel. Fennel tea 3 times daily
Dilution: Use essences 2½% in massage. 10 drops in 2 tsp (7ml/¼fl oz) vegetable oil
Effect: Toxin removal and circulation stimulation is achieved by the water, fennel tea (natural diuretic) and rosemary, juniper and cypress. Fennel and geranium also act on the hormone levels which contribute to cellulite

Ailment: **Chilblains**
Treatment: Usually the result of poor circulation (and vitamin and mineral deficiency). Massage with stimulating, anti-inflammatory oils is indicated. An ointment or cream of these oils can be applied. If painful and itching, lavender and marjoram are indicated. Lemon and rosemary are also indicated. Garlic, vitamin and mineral supplements should also be considered
Effect: Massage and regular application of the oils in dilution should prevent the onset of chilblains. Circulation stimulation using these oils should help clear them up

Ailment: **Colds**

Treatment: The viral infection which causes colds often gives rise to secondary bacterial infections. The anti-viral and anti-bacterial nature of essences such as eucalyptus, tea-tree and thyme are particularly indicated. Pine, cinnamon, cypress and sandalwood are also of use, and lavender promotes sleep and recovery generally. Vitamin C should be taken in high doses (up to 5g daily of a buffered low acid formula) and plenty of pure water consumed. Aromatic baths and massage with these oils may also help. Cypress is indicated for excessive mucus production
Dilution: Inhalations: 1 drop eucalyptus; 2 drops thyme; 3 drops tea-tree; 2 drops cinnamon; 2 drops pine; or 1 pinch black pepper; 1 drop cedarwood; 1 drop peppermint; 3 drops rosemary
Effect: The inhalations act on the invading microbes by the heat of the steam and the action of the essences, which have an antiseptic, expectorant and decongestant action. Sandalwood is especially useful for sore throats and loss of voice (diluted 5% and rubbed in throat externally). Vitamin C, if taken at the beginning (500mg every 2 hours) can prevent the cold developing

Ailment: **Cold sores/herpes**
Treatment: Apply neat lavender or tea-tree essences to the blister at first onset. If cold sore has emptied, dab area with the following blend, and alternate with the application of neat lavender if no immediate relief is forthcoming. Diet and life-style should be examined as supplements may be contributory elements
Dilution: 5ml (1 tsp) alcohol; 2 drops bergamot; 2 drops eucalyptus; 2 drops tea-tree/chamomile
Effect: This will soothe the blister, clean the site antiseptically and promote speedy healing, reducing the likelihood of scarring

Ailment: **Constipation**

Treatment: Massaging the abdomen in a clockwise motion, by aromatherapist or the sufferer, can bring great relief by stimulating the peristaltic action of the gut. Rosemary and fennel aid and stimulate digestion. Marjoram and lavender's anti-spasmodic action is also indicated. Dietary fibre may be lacking: fresh fruit and vegetables and water and adequate exercise

Dilution: 2½% in massage

Effect: Aromatherapy massage will help release the stress which often contributes to this problem. The abdominal massage mimics the peristaltic action, bringing great relief. Diet is a very important consideration here

Ailment: **Cystitis**

Treatment: Anti-bacterial, anti-inflammatory essences, should be used in sitz baths, aromatic baths and massage. Tea-tree pessaries are very effective. Sandalwood, bergamot and chamomile can be added to aromatic baths, the latter can be used in sitz baths with tea-tree, and in hot compresses on the lower abdomen when acute pain is present. Live yoghurt or acidophilus capsules are recommended, and drink plenty of pure water and chamomile tea

Dilution: Sitz baths: 1¼%; Aromatic baths: 10 drops in 2 tsp (7ml/¼fl oz) oil

Effect: This infection often attacks when stress is acute, thus aromatherapy will help prevent its onset. Massage with these essences will act on the bacteria causing inflammation of the bladder. Wearing loose-fitting clothes and cotton underwear is also recommended

Ailment: **Fatigue**

Treatment: Prolonged fatigue may be due to high stress levels, vitamin and mineral deficiency, poor diet, lack of exercise, toxic system – all of which need to be assessed. Harmonizing and stimulating oils are usually indicated, such as peppermint, rosemary, geranium, bergamot, clove, nutmeg and thyme – used in baths and massage

Dilution: No more than 2 drops of thyme, clove and nutmeg should be used in the bath, and 1 drop of peppermint

Effect: The oils have a naturally revitalizing effect without the harmful side-effects artificial stimulants such as coffee, tea, sugar, cigarettes, alcohol or drugs impart. Massage with essences relieves mental and physical tension which drains energy. The harmonizing action of oils such as bergamot and geranium balance the system, redirecting lost or diverted energy

Ailment: **Fever**

Treatment: Part of the natural healing process may involve 'sweating it out' – as the higher body temperature fights infection. If the temperature needs to be reduced, tepid sponging or cold compresses can be used – peppermint, eucalyptus, bergamot and lavender are indicated. If the subject is strong enough, a lukewarm bath can also be used with essences. Drink plenty of pure water to help cool and detoxify the system

Dilution: Tepid sponging – 1 drop of peppermint and 5 drops of lavender in 2 pints (40fl oz) lukewarm water. Compress – 1 drop eucalyptus or 1 drop of peppermint with 2 drops of bergamot

Effect: The antiseptic nature of these essences, as well as their cooling effect, will help combat the infection and reduce the temperature

NOTE: Always consult a doctor in cases of high temperatures, especially for children

Ailment: **Flatulence**

Many essences help expel excess gas from the digestive system. Used in massage of the abdomen, the clockwise circular motion will bring relief. Dietary changes may be indicated, and live yoghurt or acidophilus capsules and fennel tea are useful.

Treatment: Oils include aniseed, tangerine,

mandarin, nutmeg, thyme, spearmint, peppermint, parsley, fennel, caraway and cinnamon

Dilution: In 2½% massage

Effect: Will help the expulsion of excess gas from the digestive system, reducing abdominal bloating and discomfort

Ailment: **Headaches**

Treatment: Lavender applied to the temples or in a cold compress on the forehead or back of neck. Inhaling peppermint may also help – either with or without lavender. Neroli, rosemary and eucalyptus can also bring relief – the latter two used in inhalation for sinusitis headache due to congestion. Massage relieves headaches brought on by tension, especially muscular tension in the neck and shoulder area. Shiatsu points (governing vessel 21–24 and others – see shiatsu section) can be worked upon quickly and effectively. Lack of water or a toxic system may also cause headaches – drink a large glass of pure water. For regular or constant headaches, diet and life-style should be examined

Dilution: Undiluted 2 drops for compress. 1 drop for compress. 5 drops lavender, 2 eucalyptus, 3 rosemary

Effect: Lavender and peppermint have a strong analgesic action, and rosemary, eucalyptus and peppermint have a very cleansing stimulating effect. Lavender and neroli are particularly indicated for tension headaches

This will help cleanse the system and relieve the pain. Lack of salt, calcium or food allergies may also cause headaches

Ailment: **Hypertension (high blood-pressure)**

Treatment: Regular massage with lavender, ylang ylang, marjoram and neroli is particularly indicated. Using bergamot, frankincense, chamomile, fennel, orange, juniper and lemon will help cleanse the system and

uplift the spirit. Aromatic baths will also help, and learning a form of relaxation, deep breathing, meditation will greatly benefit the sufferer

NOTE: In the case of very high blood-pressure – medical advice should be sought before massage is used

Dilution: 2½% in massage

Effect: Aromatherapy treatment can dramatically reduce high blood-pressure. Using massage with sedative properties helps reduce the high stress levels and promotes the ability to relax. Ylang ylang has a specific action on tachycardia (over rapid heart beat) and shortness of breath, which often accompanies this condition. Diet and supplements have an important effect on reducing high blood-pressure, as does exercise. Excess weight is often a problem. Detoxifying and uplifting anti-depressant oils such as bergamot, ylang ylang, neroli and lavender may also be useful – depending on general state of mind

Ailment: **Hypotension (low blood-pressure)**

Treatment: Rosemary, black pepper, peppermint, frankincense, sage and hyssop used in massage (three of these or less) are indicated. Diet and exercise can also alter this state

Effect: Poor circulation and low blood-pressure often come together – thus stimulating essences which have a generally toning effect are indicated

Ailment: **Indigestion**

Treatment: Abdominal massage with lavender, chamomile, marjoram, clove (bud), thyme and rosemary. Hot compresses can be placed on abdomen using one of the essences. Herb teas of peppermint, fennel or chamomile will also ease discomfort

Dilution: 2½% dilution

Effect: Anti-spasmodic action will promote relaxation and aid digestion

Ailment: **Insomnia**

Treatment: Used in regular massage and aromatic baths (especially before bed), many essences promote relaxation and sleep. Lavender, neroli, chamomile, clary sage, sandalwood and frankincense can be used, and as evaporations in the bedroom at night. Diet and exercise should be examined. Artifical stimulants such as coffee, tea, chocolate, cigarettes and alcohol may prevent sleep. Natural amino acid complexes such as h-tryptophan can also bring great relief (present in milk and bananas and in capsule form)

Dilution: 2½% in massage

Effect: Aromatherapy is particularly successful in the treatment of insomnia as it promotes relaxation, a sense of well-being and generally balances the system. Many of these essences are stress relieving, antidepressant and gently sedative. Relaxation, meditation or other forms of 'switching off' are very important

Ailment: **Mouth ulcers**

Treatment: Dry the affected area and dab tea-tree essence twice daily. Washing the mouth out with 2 drops of tea-tree and myrrh in a glass of water (add a teaspoon of sea salt and stir to dissolve; this will soothe and speed up healing). Alternatively, myrrh essence dabbed on the ulcer daily is effective. High doses of vitamin C are also indicated

Dilution: Undiluted or 4 drops of essence (2 drops of each essence) used in water as a mouthwash

Effect: Both myrrh and tea-tree are antiseptic, especially effective when mouth ulcers are due to *Candida albicans*. If ulcers are a common problem, the diet will probably lack vitamin C – which can be taken 2–10g daily

Ailment: **Nausea**

Treatment: Treatment will vary according to cause of sickness. If this is due to motion/ travel sickness, inhale peppermint essence. The citrus essences, lemon, mandarin, tangerine and orange also have a very cleansing aroma, and these are indicated if sickness is due to indigestion, over-eating or general digestive sluggishness. When emotional anxiety or tension is the cause, chamomile, lavender or neroli are indicated. These oils should be used in a light abdominal massage or in a hot compress. They can also be diffused in the sickroom if nausea is due to infection. Use a compress or gentle massage if indicated. Fennel, peppermint, spearmint and chamomile teas may also help

Dilution: Undiluted, a few drops on a tissue – or from the bottle. For the compress and massage dilute at 2½% or 2 drops in a bowl of water

Effect: The stimulating cleansing and antiseptic nature of the mints will help relieve motion sickness. The citrus essences are all carminative and generally aid digestion. Chamomile, lavender and neroli calm the nerves and aid relaxation. (Rescue remedy will also have dramatic results here!)

Ailment: **Oedema (water retention)**

Treatment: For those who are overweight, or stand on their feet continually, puffy ankles can be a regular problem. Circulation stimulants such as rosemary and juniper can help. Massage, working up the leg, helps relieve excess fluid build up, while specific lymphatic drainage points can be used in the massage, using reflexology and shiatsu points. When the system is toxic, oils such as cypress, fennel, juniper and lemon will help the system detoxify itself. Geranium is useful for cellulite and water retention. Regular exercise and lying with the legs raised above the head will help

Dilution: at 2½% in massage

Effect: The rubefacient properties of rosemary and juniper will stimulate the circulation and help remove the excess lymph. Specific points in reflexology and shiatsu help the lymphatic system to function properly by stimulating the lymph glands and blood and lymph circulation

Ailment: **Palpitations (tachycardia)**
Treatment: The most useful essence for this is ylang ylang – used in regular massage treatment. If nervous anxiety or shock have triggered off this reaction, other essences can also be used which soothe and calm – chamomile, lavender, neroli and petitgrain. Diet and general life-style should also be considered. Aromatic baths can be added to the daily routine to reduce stress levels
Dilution: 2½% in massage. For baths up to 10 drops diluted in 2 tsp (7ml/¼fl oz) of vegetable oil
Effect: Regular massage has a dramatic effect on reducing high blood-pressure, and palpitations respond dramatically well too. Diet and general life-style may contribute to the state leading to palpitations. Reduced stress levels, relaxing regularly and gentle exercise may all help

Ailment: **Shingles**
Treatment: Supplements are very important here. Bergamot, eucalyptus, geranium and tea-tree are indicated. For small painful areas of blisters apply with cotton-bud or soft brush. For larger areas, dilute in alcohol and add to baths. When the rash has healed, but pain is still present, continue the use of aromatic baths, but use lavender, bergamot and chamomile
Dilution: Small areas: ⅓ eucalyptus, bergamot and tea-tree undiluted. Large areas: 60ml (2fl oz/¼ cup) alcohol, 20 drops of each of the above. Baths: 2 drops eucalyptus, 6 drops bergamot, 2 drops tea-tree; or 4 drops lavender, 5 drops bergamot, 1 drop chamomile in 2 tsp (7ml/¼fl oz) vegetable oil

Effect: The oils indicated for small and large areas help ease the pain, reduce the blisters and have a generally anti-viral action. The state of mind is also helped. When used in aromatic baths lavender is a general tonic for those who are convalescing. It also has an analgesic action; the bergamot an astringent, anti-depressant action; and the chamomile is soothing

Ailment: **Sinusitis**
Treatment: This may be due to infection and inflammation of the nasal cavaties, or general congestion due to a respiratory infection. Use inhalations as required, and diffuse essences in bedroom at night. Use the shiatsu points on the face and points in reflexology
Dilution: 1 drop peppermint, 2 drops pine, 2 drops eucalyptus, 2 drops lemon, 3 drops tea-tree; or, 1 drop thyme, 2 drops sage, 3 drops cypress, 2 drops eucalyptus, 3 drops tea-tree (half dose if too strong)
Effect: These oils are antiseptic, decongestant and expectorant. They will help fight the infection, and relieve the congestion. The shiatsu and reflexology points will dramatically relieve the pressure on the sinuses

Ailment: **Thrush**
Antifungal essences such as tea-tree and lavender are indicated. Tea-tree pessaries or cream can be used. Three drops of tea-tree can be applied to tampons and used accordingly. Aromatic and sitz baths containing lavender, bergamot and tea-tree may be used. Massage regularly using those oils – and diet should be closely examined for possible wheat, sugar or yeast allergy. If thrush occurs after the use of antibiotics, live yoghurt or acidophilus capsules are highly recommended
Dilution: 5–10 drops in 2 tsp (7ml/¼fl oz) of vegetable oil. 2½% massage
Effect: These will act on *Candida albicans*

which may have become over populated due to the upset in balance of the intestinal flora that stress, allergies or antibiotics may have caused. These often kill off the 'friendly' intestinal bacteria which then enables candida to over populate. The uplifting essences – lavender and bergamot – will help lift the spirits. When we become depressed the immune system becomes less effective allowing candida or other infections to invade the system. The acidophilus capsules contain the 'friendly' intestinal flora needed to redress the balance

Ailment: **Toothache**
Treatment: Place clove essence on a piece of wool and rub around the painful area of the tooth or gum. If there is a cavity, apply clove essence to cotton wool and place in the cavity. If the tooth is cracked, or the area clearly infected, drip the essence directly into the area. Reapply once if necessary (seek advice of dentist if problem persists). If there is an abscess, use tea-tree essence applied neat to the area very regularly. A hot compress of chamomile and lavender will also help (**adults only**)
Dilution: Undiluted, 1 drop on cotton wool. 1–2 drops for each compress
Effect: Clove oil has a local anaesthetic antiseptic action which will numb the pain and help cleanse the infected area. Lavender and chamomile compress will help ease the pain and draw the pus to the surface – speeding up the healing process. Tea-tree also has strong antiseptic properties

Ailment: **Verrucae and warts**
Treatment: Apply lemon or tea-tree to the area, or on plaster, and keep plaster on area until the area has been cleared. Reapply daily. Dietary supplements such as garlic, vitamins C and E may also be indicated
Dilution: Neat – one drop for each application
Effect: The anti-viral, anti-fungal effect of both essences should reduce the area until the infection disappears. This may take a week or a few months, but it will often work

PROBLEMS RELATING TO MENSTRUATION
Ailment: **Amenorrhoea**
Treatment: Absence of or scanty menstruation can be helped by emmenagogue essential oils. First it is important to ensure the period has not ceased due to pregnancy before using these oils. These should not be used by those with heavy flow, as this may be increased. Use massage and aromatic baths. Consider diet and life-style
Dilution: Use chamomile, sage, clary sage, geranium, hyssop, fennel at 2½%
Effect: These emmenagogue oils are oestrogen stimulants and can thus promote normal flow at this time. Stress alleviation by aromatherapy can also help regulate the menses

Ailment: **Dysmenorrhoea**
Treatment: For those who have an abnormally heavy flow, the following oils should be used in massage and aromatic baths. Diet may be particularly important here – as supplements such as a natural mineral complex with iron may be needed
Dilution: Cypress, geranium and rose at 2½%
Effect: These have a regulating normalizing effect. Anaemia can result and exacerbate the condition, thus iron supplements may be very important. The cypress and geranium have an astringent effect

Ailment: **Hot flushes**
Treatment: One of the more embarrassing effects for some during the menopausal period can be greatly relieved by geranium and rose, used in aromatic baths and massage. Chamomile, lavender, neroli, petitgrain and jasmine, clary sage, sandalwood and ylang ylang can also be helpful

Dilution: Used at 2½% in massage and 5–10 drops in 2 tsp (7ml/¼fl oz) of vegetable oil in a bath
Effect: The soothing and regulating action is important, as is the uplifting anti-depressant effect. Many suffer stress tension and lack of self confidence at this time. Massage with these oils can nurture and relax, which helps reduce the incidence of hot flushes. The oestrogen stimulating action of some oils can also be helpful

Ailment: **Mastitis**
Treatment: Warm compresses using lavender, clary sage, chamomile, geranium or rose are indicated. Massage can help stimulate lymph flow. Peppermint essence will cool
Dilution: 1–2 drops in warm water
Effect: These oils have an analgesic, soothing and regulating effect. The drawing action of the heat and the circulation stimulation in massage will help ease congestion

Ailment: **Period pains**
Treatment: Gentle massage over the lower back and abdomen with clary sage, marjoram and lavender can produce dramatic results. Hot compresses with these oils can also help. Melissa may also be used
Dilution: 2½% in massage and 1–2 drops clary sage in hot compresses
Effect: These oils have a strong antispasmodic, analgesic effect which helps relieve uterine spasm thus easing pain. These oils also have a soothing and uplifting emotional effect

Ailment: **Pre-menstrual tension (PMT)**
Treatment: At least 500mg of evening primrose oil should be taken daily, especially the week before the period. Massage treatment with lavender, neroli, petitgrain, geranium, rose and others will help. Aromatic baths also
Dilution: 2½% in massage and 5–10 drops in a bath in 2 tsp (7ml/¼fl oz) vegetable oil
Effect: It is particularly important to use the oils the woman is most drawn to. The tension is greatly alleviated by the supportive relaxing massage which will also help relieve depression

NOTE: Where many essences are recommended for specific complaints do not attempt to include every one in a specific combination. Many essences are extremely useful when used by themselves. A combination of up to five essences may be used, but it is not recommended to use more in any one blend, as they may then have a weaker effect. Generally two or three essences make a useful combination.

SKIN CONDITIONS

Skin conditions will benefit from drinking plenty of mineral (or reverse osmosis or distilled) water. This will help cleanse the system and flush the toxins that can cause skin problems. A good diet is also extremely important. Dietary analysis may be useful to ensure there is adequate intake of vitamins, minerals, and dietary fibre. Foods high in refined sugars, saturated fats and artificial additives should be avoided as much as possible. Foods rich in vitamins C,E,A and iron – such as fresh fruit and raw vegetables and plenty of pure water – should be consumed daily. Coffee, tea and alcohol should be avoided or kept to a minimum. These are recommendations which will promote general health and well-being. For most people, a healthy body is reflected in good skin condition.

For those with chronic skin conditions an allergy test is recommended. A short fast may be helpful to eliminate a toxin build-up. This must be considered carefully with your natural health therapist, as it is inadvisable in certain cases (consult your doctor if unsure). Avoid facial products containing harsh synthetic perfumes and other additives. These may exacerbate rather than ease the skin condition.

SKIN CONDITIONS

Condition: **Acne**

Treatment: Diet is a very important part of treatment and vitamin and mineral supplements can be of great benefit (vitamins A,B,C,E, evening primrose capsules, garlic, zinc – consult your nearest natural health therapist). Use a facial steam with essences 1 –2 times a week. Use lavender, bergamot and geranium. Wheatgerm and avocado oils should be added to treatment oils, creams and lotions. Massage treatment should be used regularly (once a week) to help stimulate toxin removal, and reduce stress levels. Aromatic baths should also be used regularly. Rosemary, cypress, chamomile, juniper, patchouli, sandalwood and eucalyptus can all be useful. Neroli, patchouli and lavender should be used in a night cream as skin condition improves. Evening primrose applied externally (used in massage) can be a useful addition

Dilution: To a bowl of steaming water add: lavender 4 drops, bergamot 5 drops, geranium 3 drops. These oils can also be added to facial massage oils, creams and lotions at 1%. Use neroli, patchouli, lavender and evening primrose at 5% dilution for night cream and massage.

Effect: The cleansing antiseptic action will help cleanse the skin and draw infection to the surface. The uplifting anti-depressant action of lavender and bergamot will help relieve the stress caused by and exacerbating to the skin condition. The astringent action of bergamot will help close the pores, and geranium can help balance the sebum. The addition of avocado and wheatgerm will generally assist due to the levels of vitamins E and A. Neroli, lavender and patchouli will encourage skin growth and help reduce scarring

Condition: **Blackheads**
Treatment: Use aromatic steaming facial once a week. Hot compresses can be applied to specific areas – exfoliating 2–3 times a week is also helpful. Splash face with cold water after cleansing with heat, to help close the pores. Use facial creams and toners with the oils
Dilution: 3 drops lemon, 3 drops cypress, 4 drops geranium in a bowl of steaming water
Effect: These oils have an astringent detoxifying effect that will help rid the pores of the excess sebum

Condition: **Dry skin**
Treatment: Add geranium, lavender, sandalwood, patchouli or ylang ylang to a base oil including evening primrose and avocado. Or add to 50ml of pure non-lanolin face cream (preferably with vitamin E)
Dilution: 2 drops geranium, 8 drops lavender, 8 drops sandalwood, 4 drops ylang ylang, 3 drops patchouli in 10ml (¼fl oz/2 tsp) base, 5ml avocado, plus evening primrose
Effect: This is a generally revitalizing and balancing blend which can be altered to suit personal preference. (Do not use more than 25 drops of essential oil in a 50ml base)

Condition: **Eczema**
Treatment: Massage, aromatic baths and dietary advice should again be used. Calendula cream and rescue remedy cream can also help ease the irritation and inflammation. Chamomile, yarrow, sandalwood and patchouli are indicated. Bergamot, neroli, lavender and melissa can also help. Chamomile and melissa can be a useful combination in skin cream for inflamed sore areas. Evening primrose, avocado and jojoba make particularly useful additions to massage and treatment oils. If the eczema condition

becomes more irritating with an oil-based treatment, use natural creams, gels and lotions as your base
Dilution: Use oils at 1%
Effect: These have an anti-inflammatory action. The astringent nature of bergamot, and the soothing action (at 1%) of melissa and chamomile make these useful additions. Evening primrose helps combat the inflammation, and all three help nourish the dry skin

Condition: **Oily skin**
Treatment: Add tea-tree, cypress, lemon and geranium to a light cream base or vegetable oil (such as grapeseed). Also use a facial steam 1–2 times a week with the oils. A compress may be useful once a week, plus regular exfoliation and the use of astringent toners
Dilution: 6 drops tea-tree, 9 drops cypress, 5 drops lemon, 5 drops geranium in 50ml (2fl oz/¼ cup) base oil or cream
Effect: These oils have a detoxifying astringent effect (as for blackheads)

Condition: **Psoriasis**
Treatment: Generally a very stress-related condition. Massage treatment is indicated with rich emollient oils such as avocado, wheatgerm, evening primrose and jojoba. Bergamot, peppermint and eucalyptus can help, as can chamomile and yarrow. Natural exfoliating agents can help remove scaly, dead skin cells. Diet and supplements are also very important here
Dilution: Use vegetable oils at 5%. Use essences at 1% in massage, creams and lotions
Effect: While psoriasis is difficult to cure, massage with nourishing blends and stress-relieving essences often improves the condition. The cooling astringent properties of bergamot, eucalyptus and peppermint can reduce redness, while chamomile and yarrow can have an anti-inflammatory effect

Condition: **Sensitive skin**
Treatment: Use the essences which are particularly gentle and extremely unlikely to cause any reaction (even to the most sensitive of skin): neroli, rosewood, rose and patchouli. Avoid all products which are highly perfumed and synthetic
Dilution: Use oils at 1%. 3 drops rose (optional), 5 drops neroli, 9 drops rosewood, 3 drops patchouli in 50ml of cream or base oil
Effect: A gently nourishing revitalizing combination

Condition: **Spots**
Treatment: For infected pores apply tea-tree, having cleansed the area. Use toner for oily skins (see recipe section) and exfoliate regularly. Tea-tree cream is also useful, as is rescue cream for painful spots. For the frequent sufferer, consider diet, supplements and drink plenty of pure water
Dilution: Undiluted 1 drop
Effect: The antiseptic action will act upon any infection and thus promote healing

HAIR AND SCALP PROBLEMS

The following recommendations are to be used in a base oil of 50ml (2fl oz/¼ cup). Shake blend before use. The blend should be massaged through the hair into the scalp with the fingertips. It should then be left on for 30 minutes, unless otherwise directed. To shampoo out, **apply shampoo first** before the water, otherwise the oil will be difficult to wash out properly.

Condition: **Dandruff**
Treatment: Massage blend thoroughly into the scalp. Leave on for 1 hour
Dilution: 5 drops lavender, 8 drops rosemary, 8 drops tea-tree, 4 drops cedarwood = 25 drops
Effect: Dandruff occurs due to Candida albicans (yeast infection). This blend's antispetic, anti-fungal action can help dramatically

Condition: **Dry hair**
Treatment: Massage blend into hair, covering the dry ends as well as the scalp
Dilution: 10 drops sandalwood, 10 drops rosewood, 5 drops ylang ylang = 25 drops
Effect: Will help recondition the hair

Condition: **Hair lice**
Treatment: Massage blend thoroughly throughout hair and scalp. Leave on for minimum 1 hour under cling film/shower cap, or overnight if possible. Repeat treatment 4 times over two days. Wash all bedlinen, hats and clothes
Dilution: 20 drops geranium, 40 drops bergamot, 20 drops lavender, 20 drops tea-tree = 100 drops, in 100ml (4fl oz/½ cup) vegetable oil (5%)
Effect: The length of time over which the procedure is repeated is important. This helps ensure that the eggs as well as the insects are killed

Condition: **Oily hair**
Treatment: Massage blend into scalp
Dilution: 5 drops lemon, 10 drops juniper, 10 drops cedarwood = 25 drops
Effect: These have an astringent effect on excess sebum production

ESSENTIAL IDEAS

The use of essential ideas is as limitless as the versatility of the therapeutic actions they impart. Discovering your own methods of using the oils in the home is all part of the delights they have to offer. Here are some suggestions:

PERFUME
Our choice of perfume is invariably a reflection of individual character. Modern-day, mass-produced synthetic products are not to everyone's taste. Many people are allergic to the chemicals used. The essential oils can be used effectively to create a perfume to your own personal specifications. As the oils impart actions, they can affect the mood of the wearer and those around her.

Use jojoba oil or beeswax as a base and experiment a little, it will be well worth the effort.

SCENTING CLOTHES
Why not impart a wonderful, personal aroma to your clothes.
• Sprinkle a few drops of essence on draw liners, on handkerchiefs or tissues, and place among clothes.
• Add a few drops of essence to the finishing rinse for clothes, towels and bedlinen.
• Sprinkle a few drops on bedlinen when making the bed.
NOTE: Essential oils can stain delicate material, use with care.

SCENTING YOUR HAIR
Add a few drops of your favourite essence to the finishing rinse, or conditioning treatment.

NATURAL AIR FRESHENER
A natural, ozone friendly and anti-microbial spray can be used wherever and whenever desired. Add 10% of the essences to a plant spray or similar atomizer containing water. Shake before use.

Add essence to pot-pourri to lengthen its life, strengthen its scent and personalize the aroma. Sprinkle a few drops of essence on the carpet when vacuuming to freshen the carpet and scent the room.

INSECT/PET REPELLENT
Essences such as geranium, eucalyptus, lavender and peppermint are strong insect repellents. They can be added to cream or sprayed regularly to deter anything from mosquitoes to moths. A few drops of juniper can be added when washing dogs to help remove and prevent tics and fleas.

Spraying these oils on areas where pets are a nuisance can help deter fouling in unwanted places!

CULINARY USE
The infused oils or vinegars can be used in cooking and salad dressing. Add a few drops of orange essence to your mulled wine recipe to impart an extra fruity flavour. Lemon and orange essence can add a lovely natural flavour to cakes and biscuits, and are a healthy alternative to artifical additives. A few drops of peppermint essence can be used for peppermint cream recipes.

NOTE PAPER
Keep a tissue with a few drops of essence with your note paper to impart your own favourite scent.

RECIPES

AN INFUSED OIL

This is a simple and enjoyable method of using the essential oils the herbs and flowers in your garden have to offer. The floral or herbal oil which will result from this process can be used in cookery or aromatherapy.

Take a sterile, wide-mouthed jar and fill it about one third full of petals, or other plant material. Fill the jar to the brim with a clear vegetable oil such as sesame, soya or grapeseed oil. Screw the top on tightly (excluding as much air as possible to prevent oxidation turning the mixture rancid). Place the jar in the airing cupboard, next to the Aga, or on the window-sill if the sun is shining. When the petals or leaves turn brown and begin to look 'spent', remove them and replace with fresh stock. Repeat this process until the oil smells strong enough. Strain the mixture when ready, and decant. Stored in a cool, dark place, the infused oil will last for two to three months.

If an infused oil is required urgently, the above process can be speeded up by heating the oil and plant material. Place the jar on a piece of circular material (in a saucepan) to prevent it from cracking, and simmer the contents until the plant material needs replacing. This method will produce a lesser quality infused oil.

Infused oils may be used therapeutically in massage, and can be especially useful as a gentle blend for use on babies and children. They can make a pleasant addition to a bath, and can be added to cream recipes for additional therapeutic effect. Comfrey and calendula oil are infused oils.

BATH OILS

Points to remember:

1 DO NOT use more than 10 drops of essential oil. 5 drops will often be sufficient.

2 DO NOT use more than 1 drop of peppermint or eucalyptus in your bath, as their menthol constituents are extremely strong.

3 Dilute essential oils before use, as directed:

5 drops to 1 tsp (5ml) oil

10 drops to 2 tsp (10ml) oil.

4 You can also add a naturally based bath foam if desired. (This may also help clean the bath after use.)

5 Do not leave bottles of essence on the side of plastic baths, as any neat essence may mark.

BATH OILS (*not for those with sensitive skins)

Type: **Gently sedative, sleep-inducing and stress relieving.** (Evening use only)

Effect: These oils will relieve stress and tension, and help the mind and body to unwind and 'switch off'. Frankincense, sandalwood, rosewood, mandarin, rose and vetiver may also be used

Dilution: Lavender 7 drops, marjoram 3 drops = 10 drops; bergamot 3 drops, lavender 5 drops = 8 drops; OR chamomile 2 drops, lavender 7 drops, neroli 1 drop = 10 drops; clary sage 3 drops, lavender 6 drops = 9 drops; mandarin 4 drops, neroli 2 drops = 6 drops

Type: **Refreshing, stimulating (counteracting tiredness)**

Effect: These blends will help stimulate the whole system. They will have a refreshing effect, stimulating the circulation – reviving a tired body too. Other stimulants include peppermint, eucalyptus, juniper, aniseed and sage

Dilution: Tangerine 4 drops, lemon 1 drop, rosemary 3 drops = 8 drops; rosemary 3 drops, geranium 4 drops = 7 drops; OR *thyme 2 drops, rosemary 3 drops = 5 drops; pine 3 drops, mandarin 4 drops = 7 drops; petitgrain 2 drops, rosemary 4 drops = 6 drops

Type: **Muscular aches and sprains**

Dilution: MORNING: lavender 1 drop, marjoram 2 drops, rosemary 3 drops = 6 drops; pine 3 drops, rosemary 3 drops = 6 drops; lemongrass 2 drops, coriander 2 drops, clove 2 drops = 6 drops

Effect: These oils will stimulate the circulation, helping to ease the stiffness and soothe the muscular spasm

Dilution: EVENING: clary sage 4 drops, lavender 6 drops = 10 drops; margoram 2 drops, lavender 5 drops, lemon 2 drops = 9 drops

Effect: These sedative anti-spasmodic oils will gently soothe muscular tension

Type: **Arthritis**

Dilution: MORNING: lemon 2 drops, juniper 4 drops, thyme 1 drop = 7 drops; pine 4 drops, cypress 4 drops = 8 drops

Effect: These oils will help detoxify the system by encouraging the elimination of uric acid

Dilution: EVENING: chamomile 2 drops, clary sage 4 drops = 6 drops; lavender 6 drops, cedarwood 4 drops = 10 drops

Effect: The soothing anti-inflammatory and analgesic action of most of these essences will help ease pain and promote sleep

Type: **Uplifting anti-depressants**

Effect: Geranium has an emotionally balancing effect, while bergamot and ylang ylang lift the spirits – patchouli and petitgrain also. Strongly uplifting and stress-relieving, neroli and clary sage are strong anti-depressants. Lavender and mandarin generally are a tonic for the whole system. Others include: sandalwood, frankincense, grapefruit

Dilution: MORNING: geranium 3 drops, ylang ylang 4 drops = 7 drops; bergamot 5 drops, rosemary 2 drops = 7 drops

EVENING: neroli 2 drops, lavender 6 drops = 8 drops; mandarin 4 drops, clary sage 4 drops = 8 drops

Type: **Anti-viral (immunity stimulant)**

Dilution: MORNING: *clove 2 drops, tea-

tree 4 drops, eucalyptus 1 drop = 7 drops; bergamot 5 drops, *thyme 1 drop = 6 drops
Effect: These oils stimulate the immune system, and have a strong anti-viral effect
Dilution: EVENING: bergamot 5 drops, lemon 2 drops, lavender 3 drops = 10 drops; tea-tree 3 drops, sandalwood 5 drops, frankincense 2 drops = 10 drops
Effect: These oils will have an anti-viral action, but with regulatory properties they will not stimulate the general system preventing sleep

Type: **Aphrodisiac baths**
Effect: These oils help promote relaxation of the mind and inhibitions
Dilution: ylang ylang 4 drops, neroli 2 drops = 6 drops; bergamot 6 drops, ylang ylang 4 drops = 10 drops; rose/jasmine 1 drop, neroli 2 drops = 3 drops; sandalwood 4 drops, patchouli 1 drop = 5 drops

GLOSSARY

Amenorrhoea. An absence of periods.

Analgesic. A substance which reduces or relieves pain.

Antiseptic. That which inhibits the growth of microbes such as bacteria. Most essences are antiseptic to a greater or lesser extent. Examples: tea-tree, cinnamon, clove, thyme.

Anti-spasmodic. That which relieves involuntary muscular contraction or cramp. Examples: lavender, clary sage, marjoram.

Astringent. A substance which causes the constriction of tissues, helping to reduce inflammation and pain. Examples: cedarwood, cypress, juniper.

Bach flower remedies. These are natural remedies which promote healing by having a positive action on negative states of mind or personality. They are extracted from plants and flowers (with the exception of Rock Water) by sunlight. There are 39 remedies in total. Rescue Remedy is extremely effective in cases of shock or emergency. The stock bottles can be bought in most good health food shops, or at the address given in the **'Further Reading'** section.

Bactericide. That which kills bacteria. Examples: tea-tree, eucalyptus, thyme.

Carminative. A substance which eases abdominal pain and bloating, encouraging the release of excess gas from the bowels.

Cytophylactc. A substance which stimulates skin cell growth.

Decongestant. That which relieves blockage or clogging (excess phlegm). Examples: lemon, sandalwood, cypress.

Dermal. Of the skin.

Desquamation. The peeling off or shedding of dead skin cells (massage encourages this process).

Diuretic. That which increases the flow of urine.

Dysmenorrhoea. Difficult or painful menstruation.

Emmenagogue. That which stimulates menstruation.

Emollient. A substance that has a softening or soothing effect.

Exfoliants. Substances which help peel off the layers of dead skin. Examples: oatmeal.

Expectorant. That which promotes or increases the removal of excess phlegm.

Febrifuge. That which reduces fever. Examples: eucalyptus, peppermint, bergamot.

Fungicidal. That which kills or inhibits fungal growth.

Galactagogue. That which promotes or increases the milk flow.

Holistic – (Holistic Medicine). Considering the WHOLE PERSON.

Homoeostasis. The natural balance within the system – upset by stress and shock and other factors. Maintained and assisted by complementary health therapies.

Hypertension. Abnormally high blood-pressure.

Hypotension. Abnormally low blood-pressure.

Lymphatic system. This is known as the 'drainage system' of the body. It consists of a vast network of capillary vessels connected to the veinous system which transports lymph throughout the body. The lymph contains products of metabolic waste.

Phototoxic/Photosensitization. Oils which are particularly sensitive to ultraviolet light and may cause skin pigmentation. Not to be used before going out in strong sunlight, or when using a sun bed.

Examples: all citrus oils.

Rubefacient. A substance which stimulates local circulation, causing redness to appear. Examples: rosemary, juniper, eucalyptus.

Tonic. A substance imparting a generally invigorating and beneficial effect to the whole body or specific areas.

RECOMMENDED FURTHER READING

AROMATHERAPY

Aromatherapy A-Z – Patricia Davies, Saffron Walden, C W Daniel Company Ltd

The Practise of Aromatherapy – Dr Jean Valnet, Saffron Walden, C W Daniel Company Ltd

The Art of Aromatherapy – Robert Tisserand, Saffron Walden, C W Daniel Company Ltd

The Power of Holistic Aromatherapy – Christine Stead, Javelin Books

MASSAGE

Loving Hands – Frederick Leboyer, Collins

The Complete Book of Massage – Clare Maxwell-Hudson, Dorling Kindersley

The Book of Massage – Lucinda Lidell, Ebury Press

Chinese Massage Theory – Translated by Hor Ming Lee and Gregory Whincup, Routledge and Kegan Paul Ltd

Reflexology Today – Doreen E Bayley, Thorsons

The Reflexology Workout – Stephanie Rick, Thorsons

Do-It-Yourself Shiatsu – Wataru Ohashi, Unwin Paperbacks

Acupressure Techniques, A Self-Help Guide – Dr Julian Kenyon

GENERAL

The Natural Family Doctor – Dr Andrew Stanway, Century

The Alternative Dictionary of Symptoms and Cures – Dr Caroline M Shreeve, Century

Illustrated Handbook of the Bach Flower Remedies – Philip M Chancellor

The Here's Health Magazine – The Journal of Alternative and Complementary Medicine

USEFUL ADDRESSES

(Including professional organizations only)

Culpeper Shops

Suppliers of pure essential oils and other natural high-quality products. A mail-order service is available.

London:
21 Bruton St
Berkeley Square
London W1X 7DA
Telephone 01 629 4559

8 The Market
Covent Garden
London WC2E 8RB
Telephone 01 379 6698

Bath:
28 Milsom Street
Bath BA1 1DG
Telephone (0225) 25875

Birmingham:
34 The Pavilions
High Street
Birmingham B4 7SL
Telephone 021 643 0100

Bournemouth:
1 Post Office Road
Bournemouth BH1 1DN
Telephone (0202) 27107

Brighton:
12d Meeting House Lane
Brighton BN1 1BH
Telephone (0273) 27939

Cambridge:
25 Lion Yard,
Cambridge CB2 3NA
Telephone (0223) 67370

Canterbury:
11 Marlowe Arcade
Canterbury CT1 2PT
Telephone (0227) 451121

Chester:
24 Bridge Street
Chester CH1 1NQ
Telephone (0244) 317774

Guildford:
10 Swan Lane
Guildford GU1 4EQ
Telephone (0483) 60008

Leamington Spa:
Royal Priors
Leamington CV32 4XT
Telephone (0926) 450067

Liverpool:
1 Cavern Walks
Mathew Street
Liverpool L2 6RE
Telephone 051 236 5780

Norwich:
19 Davey Place
Norwich NR2 1PJ
Telephone (0603) 619153

Oxford:
7 New Inn Hall Street
Oxford OX1 2DH
Telephone (0865) 249754

Salisbury:
25 The Maltings
Salisbury SP1 2NJ
Telephone (0722) 26159

Sheffield:
Orchard Square
Sheffield S1 2FB
Telephone (0742) 769788

York:
43 Low Petergate
York YO1 2HT
Telephone (0904) 651654

Personal shopping: all Culpeper shops are open six full days a week.

Bach Flower Remedies
The Dr Edward Bach Centre,
Mount Vernon
Sotwell
Wallingford
Oxon OX10 0PZ

Equipment Suppliers
Massage couches
New Concept
(Dept H)
Darsham
Saxmunden
Suffolk 1P17 3QN

Marshcouch
36 Glebe Close
Hemel Hempstead
Herts HP3 9FA

Herbal Medicine
National Institute of Medical Herbalists
41 Hatherley Road
Winchester
Hampshire SO22 6RR

Reflexology
Association of Reflexologists
Slaters
14 Willow End
London N20 8EP

British Reflexology Association
Monks Orchard
Whitbourne
Worcester WR6 5RB

Shiatsu
Shiatsu Society
19 Cangside Park
Kilbarchan
Renfrewshire PA10 2EP

Touch for Health
Brian H Butler BA
Touch for Health
Foundation Faculty Member
39 Browns Road
Surbiton
Surrey KT5 8ST

The Touch for Health Foundation
1174 North Lake Avenue
Pasadena
California
91104 USA

General
Council for Complementary and Alternative
Medicine
Suite 1
19A Cavendish Square
London W1M 9AD

INDEX

ACKNOWLEDGEMENTS

There are many people I would like to thank for helping to make this book, and many other things, possible. My particular thanks go to Maria Ball, for taking a risk and keeping an eye on me, and to all those I met at the Raworth Centre in Surrey where I trained. To Mike Dowling, Maria Ball and Robert Tisserand for a wonderful training, and to Mike again (also of 'Good Scents' in Sussex) for reading through the initial draft and for his valued advice. To Ann Currie and Josie Remzie for burning the midnight oil. To Ilene Stevenson for her helpful clarification of the reflexology section. To Robert and Sharon Sheargold for their financial advice and friendly encouragement. To the *Here's Health* magazine and the Enterprise Allowance Scheme for giving me such a great start. To Ian and Diana Thomas, for their sponsorship, support and patient advice.

I would also like to thank those who were instrumental in hastening my return to good health and for introducing me to complementary therapies, for which I am enternally grateful.

To my very special family – for everything. To Dorothy Baker and all those at the Wei Clinic in Bury St Edmunds. To Fred and Sarah Dale, Dave Goodey and Jean and Peter Marshal.

On a penultimate note, thanks go to all my clients, whose trust, enthusiasm and encouragement have meant a great deal to me.

Finally, this book is dedicated to my family, and all those who are about to discover complementary medicine for themselves.